An Introduction to Clinical Trials

T0177575

An Introduction to Clinical Trials

Jonathan A. Cook

Associate Professor, Centre for Statistic in Medicine, Oxford, UK

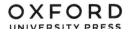

OXFORD
UNIVERSITY PRESS

OXFORD
UNIVERSITY PRESS

Great Clarendon Street, Oxford, OX2 6DP,
United Kingdom

Oxford University Press is a department of the University of Oxford.
It furthers the University's objective of excellence in research, scholarship,
and education by publishing worldwide. Oxford is a registered trade mark of
Oxford University Press in the UK and in certain other countries

Published in the United States of America by Oxford University Press
198 Madison Avenue, New York, NY 10016, United States of America

British Library Cataloguing in Publication Data

Data available

Library of Congress Control Number: 2023935555

ISBN 978–0–19–888523–8

DOI: 10.1093/med/9780198885238.001.0001

Printed in the UK by
Ashford Colour Press Ltd, Gosport, Hampshire

Preface

Clinical trials are experiments on humans. The why, when, and how of clinical trials is a serious business and needs careful consideration. Conducting a clinical trial can only be justified for honourable ends. We use clinical trials to study the impact of medical treatments, to learn which treatments work, how they work, and who they benefit. Clinical trials shine light on the complex relationship between healthcare and health. Ultimately, we do this to improve the health of society through the treatment of future patients.

It is increasingly common for a clinical trial to feature in the daily news, with a study showing that a new treatment is available for this type of cancer, a vaccine for a new virus is now ready for use, or that this new treatment is better than that old one. The COVID-19 pandemic has led to clinical trials being the topic of kitchen tables. Sadly, clinical trials have occasionally also been in the headlines for the wrong reasons. Some individuals have experienced significant harm due to their participation in a clinical trial. Clinical trials should not be carried out without pause for thought and due diligence.

As with any other scientific study, clinical trials ought to provide a reliable, reproducible, and fair result. However, they also involve many people. As well as numerous participants, many others will be involved in running the trial. Completing a clinical trial entails dealing with many of the challenges any project involving many individuals will face. To the scientific purist, clinical trials can be somewhat crude science, but to others, including myself, trials balance the scientific with the ethical and practical, which makes them fascinating and enjoyable to be involved with.

This book provides a short and accessible introduction to the basic principles and practices of clinical trials. It focuses mainly on randomized controlled trials as the 'ultimate' clinical trial. This book is intended for two primary audiences. First, it is for those who need to learn about clinical trials as part of their formal studies, such as a medical degree or a Master's course in one of a range of subjects relevant to clinical trials (e.g. medical statistics or epidemiology). Second, it is intended to be an accessible introduction or refresher for those who are involved in clinical trials in a professional capacity. Many people who work on clinical trials come from a range of educational and professional backgrounds—my wife came to work in trials after a degree in history. Others may have health professional backgrounds such as medicine, nursing, physiotherapy, and midwifery. As such, they may have had limited or no formal training in clinical trials before starting work in a new role. Any training they have had is likely to be of the theoretical kind, and without any practical exposure. Others often make the move from one of the laboratory sciences to working on clinical trials. Laboratory sciences are radically different in terms of study design, conduct, statistical analysis, and reporting. This book is intended to aid individuals in their professional lives to transition to working in clinical trials from other areas. Accordingly, clinical trials are defined, and the basic elements of a clinical trial considered. More generally, for readers of a range of backgrounds and stages, it is hoped that this book will help demystify some of the language used in this area. The underlying scientific and statistical concepts of clinical trials are presented. Furthermore, it will allow an entry point to the vast, and growing clinical trial literature.

Part of the inspiration for this book has come from my personal involvement in teaching and organizing an annual course on randomized trials. Participants often request a recommended introductory book. Many books on clinical trials exist, a number of which address the topic well, and in far greater detail than is possible here. Many others address specific aspects of clinical trials well. However, none have felt quite right to recommend as a short, accessible introduction to clinical trials. It is hoped this book will address this gap.

Another motivation has been my immersion in the world of clinical trials for the last 20 years working on trials of various diseases and treatments. I've worked with many excellent colleagues from diverse backgrounds. The need to make accessible the basic concepts behind what is being done and how each role contributes has been a recurring theme. Over that time the science of clinical trials has continued to develop. Roles have become more specialized, making it difficult to get an overview and understand why things are done in a particular way. As a statistician, you are often expected to have the answers, or at least credible attempts, to questions related to the scientific rationale for different approaches and the interpretation of findings. These questions have stimulated my thinking and the desire to understand the why, what, when, and how of clinical trials. A clinical trial is a scientific wonder, but also a complex project to conduct. This book is intended to make clinical trials and the thinking and practices behind them accessible to a wide audience.

Acknowledgements

I would like to acknowledge the insights gleaned from many papers, only some of whose respective authors I am able to acknowledge through referencing in this book. Furthermore, I would like to thank Jen De Beyer, Ruth Knight, and Daniel Maughan, and the publisher's reviewers who provided helpful comments on individual chapters. I would also like to thanks colleagues who granted permission to include information from their clinical trials, and others who made their data available to researchers like me. Another source of inspiration has been the many participants and faculty members of the Centre for Statistics in Medicine's randomized trials course. I would also like to acknowledge my wife, Johanna, from whom I've nabbed various bits of clinical trials know-how. Finally, my thanks go to many colleagues past and present at the The Centre for Healthcare Randomised Trials and Health Services Research Unit at the University of Aberdeen, and the Surgical Intervention Trials Unit, the Oxford Clinical Trials Research Unit, and the Centre for Statistics in Medicine at the University of Oxford. From you I have learned lots about the reality of conducting clinical trials, and performing them in a professional (and happy) manner. Here's a toast to many more clinical trials in the years ahead.

Contents

Abbreviations

ACTT	Adaptive Covid-19 Treatment Trial
ART	Arterial Revascularisation Trial
C	control
CADTH	Canadian Agency for Drugs and Technologies in Health
CONSORT	CONsolidated Standards of Reporting Trials
COVID-19	coronavirus disease 2019
CRF	case report form
CTA	clinical trial authorization
CTIMP	clinical trial of an investigational medicinal product
CTU	Clinical Trials Unit
DSMC	Data Safety and Monitoring Committee
EMA	European Medicines Agency
EORTC	European Organisation for Research and Treatment of Cancer
EU	European Union
FDA	Food and Drug Administration
GCP	good clinical practice
GDPR	General Data Protection Regulation
HR	hazard ratio
I	intervention
ICC	intracluster correlation
ICH	International Council for Harmonisation of Technical Requirements for Pharmaceuticals for Human Use
ICON	International Collaborative for Ovarian Neoplasia
IMP	investigational medicinal product
ISIS	International Studies of Infant Survival
IST	International Stroke Trial
LEAP	Learning Early about Peanut Allergy
MACE	major adverse cardiac events
MACRO	Defining best Management for Adults with Chronic RhinOsinusitis
MAMS	multi-arm multi-stage
MHRA	Medicines and Healthcare products Regulatory Agency
MIA(IMP)	manufacturing and import authorization for an investigational medicinal product
MRC	Medical Research Council
MRI	magnetic resonance imaging
MTD	maximum tolerable dose
NHS	National Health Service

NICE	National Institute for Health and Care Excellence
NIH	National Institutes of Health
NIHR	National Institute for Health and Care Research
OR	odds ratio
PD	pharmacodynamic
PI	principal investigator
PICOTS	Population, Intervention, Control, Outcome, Timing, and Setting
PK	pharmacokinetic
QP	qualified person
RCT	randomized controlled trial
REC	research ethics committee
RECOVERY	Randomized Evaluation of Covid-19 Therapy
RR	risk ratio
SAP	statistical analysis plan
SCT	Society for Clinical Trials
SmPC	summary of product characteristics
SPIRIT	Standard Protocol Items: Recommendations for Interventional Trials
SPT	skin prick test
SUSAR	suspected unexpected serious adverse response
TIDieR	template for intervention description and replication
TMF	trial master file
TMG	Trial Management Group
TOPKAT	Total or Partial Knee Arthroplasty Trial
TSC	Trial Steering Committee
TwiCs	trials within cohorts
VEGF	vascular endothelial growth factor
VROOM	Vaccine Response On/Off Methotrexate
WHO	World Health Organization

1
What is a clinical trial?

I shall here only observe, that the result of all my experiments was, that oranges and lemons were the most effectual remedies for this distemper [scurvy] at sea.

James Lind, 1753 (1)

A simple definition

Simply put, a clinical trial can be described as a planned scientific study involving human participants which is conducted to learn about the safety and effect (e.g. 'efficacy') of a medical treatment or related care. The intention is to undertake a scientific (and objective) assessment which allows quantification of impact at least numerically and, typically, statistically. Here the word 'clinical' refers to human participants and separates out clinical trials from purely laboratory studies which focus on human tissue and cells. It also excludes animal studies (e.g. studies looking at the effect of a drug on mice). It also indicates the focus is on medical care. This includes preventative treatments (e.g. vaccination for a novel coronavirus) and diagnostic approaches (e.g. screening and use of diagnostic tests such as magnetic resonance imaging (MRI)) as well as what might first come to mind, such as the use of a novel cancer drug. In this book, reference will typically be made to 'treatments' for convenience, though clinical trials can involve various types of interventions. These include doing nothing (see Chapter 7 for a clinical trial where the intervention is not taking a drug) and its mimic, a 'placebo'; diagnostic techniques; as well as various educational, lifestyle, and preventative approaches.

The word 'trial' is not one that is particularly attractive to the uninitiated and therefore requires explanation. It needs to be emphasized that it should be understood in this context as indicating an experiment or examination, and not an ordeal of some kind. Given this, some have suggested that the term can lead to confusion (2), and that it is best avoided when describing a clinical trial to members of the public and potential participants (e.g. describing it as a 'clinical study' or a 'research study involving patients' instead). Nevertheless, the use of the term clinical trial is ubiquitous. It is increasingly used outside of academic and medical industry settings by news outlets in media items on medical breakthroughs, which commonly refer to the findings of a 'clinical trial'. Patients may well come across a clinical trial during their care. It has been estimated that as many as one in six cancer patients in the UK were involved in a clinical trial (3). Furthermore, with the growth of the conduct of clinical trials, substantial numbers of people are involved either as a participant, or in work related to them directly (such as the author of this book) or indirectly (e.g. developing or supplying medical products used in them). The name 'clinical trial' probably has more resonance today than it has ever had before.

There are a number of key attributes of a clinical trial though they come in varying forms and can have different objectives. This will be considered in more detail later in this chapter and examples of different approaches are also covered in Chapter 2. Perhaps the most critical feature of a clinical trial is that it is a planned study; this leads to a world of potential options and opportunities (providing it can be conducted according to plan). Systems can be set up, particular people can be involved in the clinical trial, and required pieces of information can be collected and assessed. This requires planning, setting-up, and work to make it happen, typically a great amount of it. An implicit feature of a clinical trial and the approach is that it is assumed that looking at multiple individuals is a useful thing to do. In other words, there is some consistency that can be achieved, and some sort of useful overview can be produced. Simply put, there is strength in numbers, and observing the impact of a treatment in a consistent manner across multiple people is informative.

Overview of the history of clinical trials

The coming of clinical trials

Most commentators agree that James Lind, a Scottish surgeon, conducted what might be viewed as the world's first proper clinical trial in 1743 on a naval ship (4). Lind planned, conducted, and reported a study on 12 selected seamen suffering from scurvy which compared potential treatments (1). He divided them up into pairs who each received one of six different remedies suggested by others to aid recovery. The six treatments with varying doses were cider, 'elixir of vitriol' (diluted sulphuric acid), vinegar, seawater, oranges and lemons, and a spice paste with barley water. He noted the 'sudden and visible good effects' from the use of oranges and lemons. Sadly, it took some time (in this case over 40 years) for the findings to be widely accepted, a fate not that unfamiliar to some who conduct clinical trials today. The concept of some sort of 'trial' of treatments conducted under a scientific basis (an 'experiment') took hold over the next 150 years through the influence of the work of Lind and many others.

The application of scientific thinking and the need for scientific experiments to assess medical treatments became much more widely accepted during the 19th century. The inadequacy of animal testing, the 'play of chance', and the potential for at least false promise from poorly conducted 'tests', if not outright harm, had become apparent through a number of infamous cases (5). Use of numerical data, beyond crude summaries of the overall state, to assess medical treatments had also begun to occur. The aforementioned concerns cumulated in a substantial number of controlled experiments of medicine being conducted around the beginning of the 20th century throughout the world (6). The need for a fair control (reference) group in order for the assessment to be useful had long been recognized (7). However, what type of control would be 'adequate' was uncertain. Allocation of the treatment to patients by 'alternation' had increasingly been in use in experiments since at least the early 19th century (8).

In the simplest form of alternation, the first patient receives one treatment ('intervention'), the second receives the other treatment ('control'), the third patient the first treatment ('intervention'), the fourth the second treatment ('control'), and so on until all the individuals have received one of the two treatments (Table 1.1). While such allocation of treatments was planned and intentional, it was also 'random' in the sense of not being determined by a doctor's preference, prognosis, or instinct, nor was it based upon the patient's condition or any other process of selection. Thus, the groups could be expected to be 'alike except in treatment' (9). However, the use of alternation suffered from one clear weakness. It was not difficult to identify the pattern, and therefore to know in advance the treatment that future patients would receive. For example, if the fifth patient was known to have received the intervention treatment, then the next (sixth) patient would receive the control. Such knowledge of future allocations could lead to undermining of the evaluation, whether due to 'our personal idiosyncrasies, consciously or unconsciously applied, or our lack of judgement' (5,10).

In 1931, the UK Medical Research Council (MRC) set up a 'therapeutic trials committee' to resolve 'the problem of securing trustworthy clinical trials of products produced by manufacturers' (11). As part of this system, the epochal MRC streptomycin trial of 107 participants, reported in 1948, led to the widespread use of controlled clinical trials, and the use of random allocation of treatment to achieve comparable groups (12). It was not the first

Table 1.1 Alternation and random allocation of two treatments (intervention and control)—example sequences

Patients in order of recruitment	Allocation under alternation	Allocation under 'simple' random allocation
1	Intervention	Intervention
2	Control	Control
3	Intervention	Control
4	Control	Control
5	Intervention	Intervention
6	Control	Control
7	Intervention	Intervention
8	Control	Intervention
9	Intervention	Control
10	Control	Intervention

Note: in its simplest form, alternation for two treatments is equivalent to giving the patients with an 'odd' number one treatment (in this case, the 'intervention' treatment) and the patients with an even number the other (the 'control' treatment). An advantage of alternation is that the groups are evenly sized even if not all of the intended patients are recruited (at most there is only a difference of one). While the simple randomization example shown here also has conveniently five patients with the intervention and five with the control treatment, this does not need to be the case. It is possible with simple randomization for all ten patients to be allocated the same treatment (i.e. all get the intervention or all get the control treatment). However, this is unlikely (1 in 500 chance given a 1:1 allocation ratio, i.e. an even chance of being in each group for each of the ten allocations). An imbalance in the numbers who receive each treatment under simple randomization in each group is quite likely (three out of four times on average).

study to 'randomize' the allocation of treatments as opposed to using a fixed sequence like alternation (5,8). Lind might even have performed randomization by casting lots or a die back in the 18th century, as the method of allocation was not recorded (1). However, the MRC streptomycin trial likely had so much impact for two main reasons. First, it identified positive findings for a common and serious condition (tuberculous) for which previous treatments had failed. Second, it was an exemplar of a well-conducted clinical trial with clear reporting of its methods and findings. It utilized several methodological approaches which would become synonymous with clinical trials. These included tailored patient eligibility criteria, implementation in multiple locations (multiple 'centres' or 'sites'), stratified randomization with concealed treatment allocation using sealed envelopes (with the allocation written on a card inside) in an order determined by random numbers (see Chapter 3 for discussion of randomization methods), defined treatments, and the use of independent assessors who were not aware of the allocation to conduct the evaluation of the outcome of patients. Furthermore, the MRC streptomycin trial came out of a system for clinical trial approval and delivery as opposed to a one-off study. It thus pointed the way to the conduct of further studies, and the value of drawing upon lessons from previous studies. In addition, an articulate statistician, Bradford Hill, who was part of the study team, was a strong, reasonable, and compelling advocate for the conduct of clinical trials (10). It was due to his influence that the use of allocation by random number was adopted in the MRC streptomycin trial. This was used to address the possibility of undermining of the comparability of the groups by those recruiting patients, something that had occurred in an earlier MRC-run clinical trial which utilized allocation by alternation (13). The MRC streptomycin trial therefore served as a model for how to conduct a clinical trial, in particular, one that used random allocation of treatments—a randomized controlled trial (RCT).

The rise of clinical trials

The number of clinical trials slowly increased over the next 20 years. From the 1950s onwards, clinical trials, and in particular RCTs, started to be used across medicine, not only for new drugs but also to evaluate existing drugs and other treatments. The use of placebo-controlled trials became more commonplace in the 1950s, such as in a large multicentre trial of an antihistamine, thonzylamine, for the treatment of the common cold, which demonstrated no benefit over the placebo control (tablets which were similarly sugar-coated and 'indistinguishable in appearance') (14). Not long after, a placebo surgery control was used in clinical trials, and this led to the abandonment of a popular operation for angina (15). The potential of the clinical trial to evaluate medical care was further demonstrated during this period by the mammoth, but also controversial, 1954 polio vaccine field trial. This landmark trial (really two studies in one) involved 1.8 million children in the US, Canada, and Finland (16). In one study involving over 400,000 children, a form of random allocation was used to determine whether the vaccine or a placebo control was to be received. The remaining participants received either the vaccine or the control according to their school grade: second graders (7–8-year-olds) received the vaccine whereas first and third graders (6–7- and 8–9-year-olds) did not. The placebo-controlled study demonstrated the vaccine was highly effective and the vaccine was quickly mass-produced and a vaccination programme established (16). By 1970, the clinical trial—and increasingly the RCT, perceived as the optimal form of it—was accepted within the medical literature as the scientific standard for evaluating drugs across a range of conditions. The use of clinical trials to address clinical questions had appeared in many areas of medical care (5). With this growing acceptance of clinical trials, more clinical trials began to appear in the subsequent decades (1970s to 1990s), steadily at first and then at an increasing pace. Clinical trials, and large RCTs in particular, began to be the vehicle by which the medical care for common and high-profile conditions such as diabetes, heart disease, and breast cancer was redefined and refined (5,12). The landmark 'mega-trial', ISIS-1, involved 16,027 patients with suspected acute myocardial infarction and demonstrated that atenolol, a beta-blocker, reduced morality. As impressive as the clinical finding was, the conduct of an RCT simultaneously in 245 centres across 14 countries and spanning six continents was perhaps more remarkable. Growth in the conduct of clinical trials continued apace into the 21st century with studies spanning all branches of medicine, to varying degrees. In oncology, clinical trials became the way to evaluate new agents and treatments; this became a legal necessity (in many countries) and the recognized and required scientific standard. More than any other area of medicine, it became de rigueur to carry out clinical trials of new cancer treatments and combinations of them, and to compare them against the existing standard of care. Collaborative groups to facilitate the conduct of such trials, such as the National Cancer Institute's Clinical Trials Cooperative Group Program in North America and the European Organisation for Research and Treatment of Cancer (EORTC) in Europe, were established in 1955 and 1962, respectively. These grew in size, influence, and productivity, making participation in clinical trials a real possibility for cancer patients in participating countries. A key driver of this growth was the provision of infrastructure to support new clinical trials, with specialist expertise in management and co-ordination, statistics, and experience of delivering clinical trials. Around the same time, the capacity of pharmaceutical companies to deliver clinical trials increased markedly, particularly in response to the impact of regulations in the US (17). Over the last 30 years clinical trials have been used to evaluate increasingly varied aspects of clinical care, not just the direct treatment, or the prevention, of disease. It is unusual for a leading medical journal not to contain the report of at least one RCT within each issue. Beyond medicine, the use of the RCT design, and the underlying scientific approach to assessment which clinical trials embody, have spread into other areas of public life and sciences, though not without controversy (18). As with medicine in general, there has been increasing recognition of the importance of patient and public perspectives in the last 20 years or so. This has correspondingly influenced the conduct of clinical trials for the better.

The statistical science of clinical trials began to develop rapidly around the 1960s onwards. Areas of interest included the statistical considerations for difference types of clinical trials, how to determine the required sample size for a clinical trial, how to randomize, and how to approach stopping a clinical trial early, along with more elaborate statistical analyses for different types of data. R.A. Fisher, the statistical pioneer, had in the 1920s provided a statistical theory to underpin the use of, and indeed the need for, random allocation (in the field of agriculture) in order to underpin statistical analyses. This likely influenced Bradford Hill and his thinking about randomization of treatments though it was only in the 1950s and onwards that the direct statistical implications of the randomization of treatment allocation were spelt out (13,19). Reflecting the academic (by no mean solely statistical) and practical challenges of clinical trials as well as the broader social and ethical issues, the Society for Clinical Trials (SCT) was founded in 1978 in the US. The SCT sought to promote and facilitate discussion related to the design and conduct of clinical trials, with the first issue of its sponsored journal, *Controlled Clinical Trials*, published in 1980. Other clinical trial-specific journals followed over time, including the SCT's re-launched journal *Clinical Trials*. A vast array of medical journals and others focused on related methodology. The medical literature now contains a huge number of articles reporting the results of clinical trials and aspects of medical research methods inspired by them.

Impact of legislation on clinical trials

The danger of untested drugs and the potential for harm had become increasingly apparent during the 19th and early 20th centuries (5). A particularly horrific and avoidable disaster was the use of thalidomide for morning sickness in the 1950s (5,20). It had originally been developed as a tranquillizer but was later promoted as a cure for nausea during pregnancy. The lack of adequate testing before being used for this purpose led to hundreds of birth defects before the drug was withdrawn from use. A twist in the story of thalidomide was that 40 years later, after a much more rigorous testing process, thalidomide would be found to be an effective treatment for myeloma. Concerns about the dangers of new drugs led to the formation of bodies such as the Food and Drug Administration (FDA) in the US, and regulations over marketing drugs elsewhere. Over the 20th century, expectations increased (to begin with, only safety had to be shown), progressing to a legal requirement in the US of evidence of efficacy as well as safety through 'adequate and controlled studies' in 1962 (5). By 1970 this was interpreted to require RCTs for new drugs (17). Similar drug regulations were mirrored in a number of other countries, leading to the formation of a worldwide clinical trials industry as pharmaceutical companies sought to demonstrate the value of new drugs across medicine. Alongside this, organizations and companies seeking to facilitate the conduct of clinical trials came into existence. The evaluation of drugs has become an elaborate and complex system from pre-clinical discovery through to final approval with clinical trials at its core (see 'Types of clinical trials' for consideration of the different types of clinical trial). More recently, further legislation in a number of countries including the US, European Union (EU) member states, and the UK has mandated the registration of certain clinical trials and making available the results once the study is complete.

With the impetus of the high standards required for drugs, clinical trials have also become the desired, if not the default, evaluative approach to compare treatment options for other kinds of treatments (such as surgery), and related aspects of medical care (e.g. new discharge policies). The burden of funding such studies, where no commercial interest exists, has been taken up by governmental agencies, international bodies such as the World Health Organization (WHO), and medical charities. However, for non-drug treatments, and to an extent 'off-label' treatments (the use of drugs for another indication other than that which it is licensed for and is stated on the labelling), it is not mandatory prior to use. The use of clinical trials is now ubiquitous across all areas of medicine. Robust controlled evaluations such as clinical trials of these other treatment options tend to occur later on in the evaluation process, and often after widespread use, if at all (15).

Ethics and clinical trials

Experimentation gone wrong

The interplay between ethical concerns and the conduct of clinical trials, particularly RCTs, was noted early on (10). Initial concerns tended to emanate from two main areas: first, whether doctors would be willing to be involved in a clinical trial given their focus on the well-being of the patient ('first do no harm'); and second, what sort of comparison group ('control') would be appropriate so as to respect the individual participant and their health. It was recognized by even the advocates of clinical trials, and RCTs most pertinently, that an ethical justification could not be presumed. A decision would need to be made on a case-by-case basis. If a study is to be conducted, the justification must rest on what is already known, what the study can achieve, and what will happen to the participants. How that might be considered from the perspective of the health professional continues to be a source of debate, particularly whether the community or the individual view is of most importance (21). A state of uncertainty, that of being in 'equipoise', has been mooted as necessary for health professionals to be able to take part in good conscience. Other commentators have emphasized more the importance of the autonomy of participants, and of individuals consenting to what will happen to them if they take part, which may be sufficient justification even if it is not perhaps optimal care in the opinion of others.

In the aftermath of the Second World War, the horrors of human abuses became more fully known through the Nuremberg trials of Nazi war criminals and those responsible for medical experiments on prisoners of war and civilians. An international standard for the conduct of 'permissible medical experiments' was needed. The Nuremberg Code's ten points outlined a number of key principles including the essential role of 'voluntary consent' and the participant's right to withdraw from the study, the need for scientific justification for the experiment, the importance of the minimization of harm, the need for careful balance of any adverse risk versus the potential benefit, and the appropriate conduct of the experiment including consideration of stopping the experiment early. A number of infamous research studies, including some clinical trials, were conducted with clear scientific rationale but with scant or no regard for the participants during the 1940s to 1970s. These took place in Australia, the UK, Canada, Sweden, and the US among other countries. Some participants were exposed to diseases (e.g. syphilis) without their knowledge or consent, or they were denied accepted medical treatment which was available before or during the study's conduct (22). In some studies, disadvantaged minority groups in society were exploited, reflecting some recognition of the pernicious nature of the studies being carried out as well as prejudiced views about the sanctity of the lives of the affected individuals. Concerns about 'unethical' practices involving a small number of contemporary studies continue to this day. Thankfully this typically relates to far less egregious forms of malpractice, though the consequences in some cases may cause great harm to the individuals concerned (23). A recent example is the TGN1412 clinical trial conducted in the UK which did not meet recognized practices regarding informed consent, presentation of relevant information for ethical approval, and of minimizing risk to participants by staggering the receipt of a new medicinal product which had never before been given to humans (23,24). Six men became seriously ill and one had to have his fingers and toes amputated.

The development of international ethical standards

The international ethics standards for medical research were further codified in the Declaration of Helsinki developed by the World Medical

Association in 1964, and subsequently revised on a number of occasions (most recently in 2013). While retaining a focus on the primacy of the patient's rights and interests, later versions were more complete and nuanced including an emphasis on the need for medical research. Protecting the needs of vulnerable groups and individuals, the need for a formal ethical review, the use of placebos, handling the informed consent process where individuals' informed consent may not be required, and the registration and reporting of clinical studies were addressed. Individual countries had started to implement their own legal frameworks and regulations, often referring to a specific version of the declaration of Helsinki (e.g. in the US the 2008 version is referred to). There was a need for international standards to harmonize regulations across countries for the conduct for clinical trials for drug approvals. This needed to reflect the nature of associated research, and the increased complexity and associated costs. This led to the development of 'good clinical practice' (GCP) specifically for clinical trials of drugs ('medicinal products') which came into effect in 1997 under the auspices of the International Conference on Harmonisation of Technical Requirements for Registration of Pharmaceuticals for Human Use (25) (known since 2015 as the International Council for Harmonisation of Technical Requirements for Pharmaceuticals for Human Use (ICH)). The ICH brought together representatives from industry and regulators from a range of countries including EU member states, the US, Canada, Japan, and also the WHO. It developed 13 core ICH-GCP principles including among other things the need for a detailed protocol and for ethical review prior to conduct. It also produced guidelines for practice going beyond these core principles into areas such as pharmacovigilance (drug safety) and statistical analyses, a process ongoing to the present day. In the EU, observing the core principles of the ICH-GCP became a legal requirement for clinical trials of drugs effective from 2004 and in the US from 2008 (26), and this has been mirrored in other countries around the world (27). Of note, EU legislation requires any clinical trials being used for approval purposes had to be conducted in accordance with the same ethical principles irrespective of where the study was conducted (28). While not legally required for many clinical trials of non-drug treatments, it is more widely viewed that other types of clinical research should also be carried out in accordance with the 'principles of GCP'. Ethical review by an 'independent' body of the research proposals has become the international standard for all clinical trials and for other medical research studies involving human participants.

Types of clinical trials

Clinical trials of drugs for regulatory approval for clinical use

There is no typical clinical trial. They vary greatly in terms of their research objectives, statistical design, data collection, outcomes, and statistical analysis. However, some broad features can be outlined. This is most easily understood in the context of the evaluation of new drugs and seeking approval for human use (e.g. to undergo assessment by a body such as the FDA in the US). Clinical trials which fall under the corresponding legislation are called trials of a 'medicinal product'; they must be set-up and conducted in a particular way. The practical implications of this are considered in Chapter 6.

Conventionally, clinical trials have been categorized according to their phase (phases 1–4). An outline of what these studies might look like is given in Table 1.2. The focus initially is on ensuring the safety of the drug and making a corresponding initial assessment. It moves towards a final

Table 1.2 Phases of drug clinical trials

Type	Phase 0	Phase 1	Phase 2	Phase 3	Phase 4
Main objective	Exploratory	Dose determination/ escalation and safety	Preliminary assessment of efficacy and safety	Confirmatory assessment of efficacy and safety	Post-marketing surveillance
Size	Circa 10–15	Circa 20–80	Circa 100–300	Circa 1000+	Unknown
Population	FIH healthy volunteers/ patients	Healthy volunteers/ patients (may be FIH)	Subset of clinical population thought to benefit	Clinical population thought to benefit	Treated population
Design	Single arm, one centre	Usually single arm, one centre	Often controlled (may be randomized), possibly multicentre	Randomized, multicentre	Typically passive, population
Control group	No	Unlikely	Maybe	Yes	No
Key outcomes	Proof of mechanism	Recommended dose/maximum tolerable dose, toxicity	Disease activity/clinical surrogate	Patient-orientated outcomes	Adverse events

FIH, first-in-human.

assessment of the clinical effect (or 'efficacy' as it is usually referred to) as the phase of the trial increases. Phase 1 trials focus on the understanding of the pharmacokinetic (PK, i.e. the impact of the body on the drug) and pharmacodynamic (PD, i.e. the impact of the drug on the body) effects of the drug. Pharmacokinetic assessments focus upon the absorption, distribution, metabolism, and excretion of the drug. Pharmacodynamic assessments look at clinical signs, functional changes, and molecular changes indicative of the drug related to the mechanism of action (the way the drug is believed to work). A key objective of a phase 1 trial is typically to identify a suitable dose for the drug that could be used in the subsequent clinical trials. Phase 2 clinical trial evaluations tend to involve an initial assessment of clinical efficacy though it may still focus on the PK and PD properties of the drug. Assessments at this phase may consider whether the drug works in the intended manner, and whether there any signs of positive clinical effect. In phase 3, the clinical trial is predominantly designed to provide a reliable answer to whether the drug works, though assessing safety remains a key area of interest. The data from phase 1–3 clinical trials are used to seek regulatory approval to use the drug in clinical practice. The gap between phase 3 and phase 4 is when regulatory approval ('marketing approval') to use the drug in clinical practice is granted. Phase 4 trials are accordingly often described as 'post-marketing' studies, and their design reflects the availability of the drug outside of a research setting. As such, phase 4 studies are less common, and typically of a less rigorous scientific nature. Conduct of each subsequent trial is conditional upon the 'success' of the preceding studies as defined by their primary objective and the absence of any preemptive safety concern.

Prior to phase 1, particularly in well-developed research areas such as oncology, a large amount of careful pre-clinical research will be carried out before embarking on the initial (typically a phase 1) clinical trial for a new drug. Despite all this careful work and increasing sophistication in drug development, most candidate drugs fail to progress fully through the evaluation to approval for human use. It has been suggested that only around 10% of potential cancer agents which are evaluated in clinical trials become medical treatments (29). To address this, a phase 0 clinical trial, to precede a phase 1 clinical trial, has been proposed. The intention is to conduct exploratory clinical research to assess the mechanism of action and potentially prepare for the later formal assessment of PKs and PDs in phase 1 and 2 trials. To date, there has been limited use of the phase 0 design.

The driver of the differences between phases in terms of the key study characteristics (i.e. its size, population, design, the use of a control group, and the main outcomes of interest) is the primary research objective of the study. This focus typically begins with an exploratory focus in phases 0 and 1, and moves through dosage assessment and safety (phase 2), to efficacy and safety (phases 2 and 3). Finally, a phase 4 study is conducted for 'post-marketing surveillance', that is, assessment of the medicinal product in clinical use. Associated outcomes used to address the corresponding objective differ accordingly, beginning in phase 0 with proof of the hypothesized mechanism of action. In phase 1 the identification of the maximum tolerable (or tolerated) dose (MTD), the highest dose which produces an acceptable level of toxicity and/or side effects, is often the focus (30). Phase 2 trial outcomes focus on evidence of disease activity or a 'clinical surrogate'. Surrogate in this sense refers to a measure which is easy to measure and is known, or at least presumed to be, related to an outcome of direct interest. Some measures of disease activity could be viewed as a surrogate for the ultimate key clinical outcome (e.g. prostate-specific antigen control in lieu of observing prostate cancer progression or mortality). Phase 3 trial outcomes tend to be more patient oriented or clinical event focused (e.g. morality). Finally, in phase 4, the focus is usually on 'rare' adverse events and which might reflect differences in the clinical usage of the drug from that for which it was initially approved.

Research designs are typically single arm in phase 0 or 1 with controlled studies and predominantly RCTs in phase 2 or 3. The size of the respective study increases as the study phase increases. Accordingly, phase 2 and 3 studies are often multicentre (i.e. they operate in multiple locations, commonly though not necessarily hospitals) in order to be able to recruit sufficient participants. The numbers presented in Table 1.2 should not be viewed as a strict rule (Chapter 5 explores how for the most common phase 3 trials samples sizes can vary greatly). Instead, they are an indication of likely scales of magnitude though this will vary according to the condition and the ease (or not) of measuring the outcomes of interest.

In terms of participants, phase 0 and 1 studies may include only healthy participants to reduce the risk of potential health problems on vulnerable patients. Phase 2–4 studies focus upon the clinical use of the drug (even if in somewhat artificial circumstances for phases 2 and 3), and therefore these are studies of patients. A positive result from a phase 3 trial (often two studies are conducted and needed) would enable an application for use in clinical practice (regulatory approval). Phase 4 trials occur after regulatory approval (e.g. by the FDA in the US, the European Medicines Agency in an EU member state, or the Medicines and Healthcare products Regulatory Agency

(MHRA) in the UK) to use and, depending upon the country, 'market' the drug. They often take the form of a passive 'surveillance' study where the focus is on rare unexpected events, which could warrant reconsideration of the use of the product. The patients from whom data are collected therefore reflect, in theory, the full range of patients who receive the drug in clinical practice. Any drug that is approved may undergo further assessment by relevant bodies (e.g. the National Institute for Health and Care Excellence (NICE) in England, and the Canadian Agency for Drugs and Technologies in Health (CADTH)) to assess whether the use of the drug offers value for money to the healthcare system and whether it should be routinely offered to relevant patients. Regulatory bodies may also have systems whereby safety concerns related to an approved drug or medical device can be raised (e.g. the yellow card system operated by the MHRA in the UK) outside of a clinical trial evaluation.

Two example clinical trials of a medicinal product

We can consider how different clinical trials can be by using two examples. An example early phase 1 trial is described in Table 1.3. This study looked at an antibody (PRX002) intended to reduce the level of a protein (α-synuclein) which previous studies had suggested was linked to progression of Parkinson's disease (31). It was the first time it was used in a human ('first-in-human'). The study involved 40 healthy volunteers to primarily assess safety and PK properties of the drug. PD properties were a secondary objective. From Figures 1.1 and 1.2, the clear impact of the differing doses on the level of the drug in blood over the follow-up period and also the rapid effect of the drug on the target protein are apparent. Given these findings, and the minor nature of the limited observed adverse events, a subsequent phase 1 trial in patients was carried out (32). This in turn led to a phase 2 study; the recently published findings from this study have sadly not borne out the promise of the phase 1 studies (33).

In contrast, an example phase 3 drug trial is described in Table 1.4 (ICON6) which looked at the use of a drug called cediranib (34). This drug is intended to inhibit vascular endothelial growth factor (VEGF) production, and has been suggested to be linked to cancer progression. The ICON6 trial looked at the safety and efficacy of this drug for women with recurrent ovarian, fallopian tube, or peritoneal cancer. The potential benefit of receiving cediranib alongside chemotherapy only, or alongside and also subsequent to it, was evaluated against having chemotherapy alone (using a placebo control). ICON6

Table 1.3 Phase 1 clinical trial of PRX002

Background	Pre-clinical and clinical evidence suggested the α-synuclein protein contributes to progression of Parkinson's disease. The PRX002 antibody was developed to target particular forms of α-synuclein
Objective	The primary objective was to evaluate the safety, tolerability, and PKs of PRX002 in healthy volunteers. Secondary and exploratory objectives assessed immunogenicity and PDs
Design	Single-centre, double-blind, placebo-controlled, single ascending dose, first-in-human, phase 1 randomized controlled trial
Population	40 healthy volunteers, age 21–58 (median 37) years, 15 men and 25 women in the US
Treatments	One of five dose levels of PRX002 or placebo via 60 min intravenous infusion
Duration	16 weeks, four screening plus 12-week follow-up
Key findings	• No serious adverse events or dose-limiting toxicity • Only mild (e.g. headache, nausea) treatment-related adverse events • Serum PRX002 exposure was proportionate to dose (Figure 1.1) • Half-life was around 18 days across doses • Dose-dependent reduction with 1 hour of administration (Figure 1.2)
Conclusions	• Serum α-synuclein level can be safely modulated using PRX002 • Further evaluation of the safety, tolerability, and PK and PD effects in patients with Parkinson's disease is warranted
Registration	ClinicalTrials.gov: NCT02095171 Subsequent clinical trials on patients with Parkinson's disease—ClinicalTrials.gov: NCT02157714 (32) and NCT03100149 (33)
Reference	Schenk DB, Koller M, Ness DK, Griffith SG, Grundman M, Zago W, et al. First-in-human assessment of PRX002, an anti-α-synuclein monoclonal antibody, in healthy volunteers. Movement Disorders. 2017;32(2):211–218

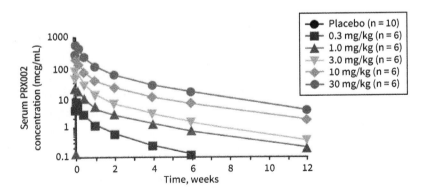

Figure 1.1 Pharmacokinetics of PRX002. Serum PRX002 concentration–time profiles after a single dose of PRX002.

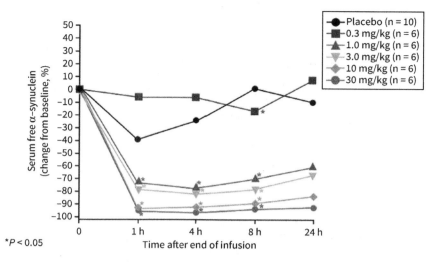

Figure 1.2 Pharmacodynamics of PRX002. Change from baseline of serum-free α-synuclein after a single dose of PRX002.

involved just under 500 women and in order to recruit the right patient group, it operated in 63 centres across five countries. Despite this, it still took over 4 years to complete recruitment. Figures 1.3 and 1.4 show the different levels of cancer progression and survival of study participants over time in the three treatments groups (arms A–C) in the study. There was statistical evidence of difference in the primary outcome, time to ovarian cancer progression, but not in overall survival (a bittersweet finding).

Clinical trials in reality

While the outlined pathway as presented in Table 1.2 is well established, it presents an increasingly artificial scheme of the evaluation of drugs and the role of clinical trials. Three key factors drive this. First, the legislation within countries related to the use of drug treatments does not proscribe the phases as indicated previously, merely the need for evidence and authorizations prior to use. In the US, the relevant legislation was amended in 1962 to require that for a new drug to be approved there had to be 'substantial evidence' of 'effectiveness' as well as 'safety'. This 'substantial evidence' was defined as coming from 'adequate and well-controlled investigations' (i.e. clinical trials). This has been typically understood to require a minimum of two clinical trials (usually RCTs) that show the drug is safe and will have the effect it purports under proposed labelled conditions of use (5). Within the EU, the original regulation

Table 1.4 Phase 3 clinical trial—ICON6

Background	Previous clinical trials have suggested that inhibitors of angiogenesis (including VEGF receptor) could lead to shrinkage of ovarian tumours and delay progression. Cediranib, an oral VEGF receptor inhibitor, seemed to reduce disease activity for different cancers. A phase 2 trial suggested similar benefit for recurrent ovarian cancer
Objective	To assess efficacy and safety of cediranib in combination with platinum-based chemotherapy and as continued maintenance treatment in patients with first relapse of platinum-sensitive ovarian cancer
Design	Multinational, multicentre, randomized placebo-controlled phase 3 trial. The trial originally had three stages: stage one was safety, stage two efficacy with a progression-free survival outcome, and the third stage concerned overall survival. The study was redesigned part way through to focus on progression-free survival as the manufacturer had discontinued the drug's development due to disappointing phase 3 clinical trial results for treatment of other cancers
Population	486 women with recurrent ovarian, fallopian tube, or peritoneal cancer requiring further chemotherapy from Australia, Canada, New Zealand, Spain, and the UK
Treatments	One of three groups: A: placebo + chemotherapy then placebo only B: cediranib 20 mg once daily + chemotherapy then placebo only C: cediranib 20 mg once daily + chemotherapy then cediranib 20 mg once daily
Study duration	49 months recruiting with median treatment and follow-up times of 8 and 20 months, respectively
Key findings	• Initial dose level of 30 mg was found to lead to toxicity in stage 1, and therefore the dose was reduced to 20 mg for the remainder of the trial • Cancer progressed in 96%, 90%, and 86% of participants in groups A, B, and C, respectively, and time to progression differed between groups (Figure 1.3) • Median time to death varied between 21 and 26 months but statistical analysis did not demonstrate a difference (Figure 1.4)
Conclusions	Addition of cediranib with and after chemotherapy prolonged time without progression of ovarian cancer but this was not shown to lead to better overall survival
Registration	ClinicalTrials.gov: NCT00532194 ISRCTN registry: ISRCTN68510403 ANZ Clinical Trials Registry: ACTRN1261000016003 Related key phase 2 trial does not appear to have been registered
Reference	Ledermann JA, Embleton AC, Raja F, Perren TJ, Jayson GC, Rustin GJS, et al. Cediranib in patients with relapsed platinum-sensitive ovarian cancer (ICON6): a randomised, double-blind, placebo-controlled phase 3 trial. Lancet. 2016;387(10023):1066–74

VEGF, vascular endothelial growth factor.

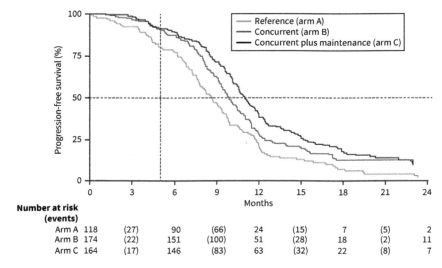

Figure 1.3 Kaplan–Meier plot of progression-free survival over 2 years.

in 1965 required 'results from clinical trials' as part of the submission to obtain approval for drugs without which no marketing could be done (35). The phases of clinical trials as indicated developed as a response to the legislation, and as such there is freedom to refine and adapt on a case-by-case basis as long as the legal requirements are ultimately met, and the regulators who act as their guardians are satisfied. Second, the time to conduct sequentially phase

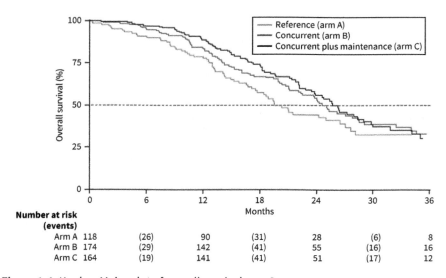

Figure 1.4 Kaplan-Meier plot of overall survival over 3 years.

1–4 clinical trials from beginning to end can take in excess of 10 years, and cost hundreds of millions of US dollars (36). As the two examples above show, in practice the evaluation path varies from drug to drug, depending upon what is already known about it, and the intended condition for which it would be used. ICON6 benefited from existing research on the candidate drug intended for other, though similar, uses; but it arguably also suffered from the absence of specific early phase work that might have been undertaken for a novel agent (and might have led to the lower dose being chosen for the phase 3 evaluation from the outset instead of being adopted partway through). The third driver of change in the evaluation process is the cost of the process of developing and bringing a new product through to clinical use which has grown massively over the last 20–30 years. This varies between jurisdictions and reflects specific evidence required for approval, and requirements related to conducting clinical trials (37). Finance influences the evaluation of drugs to the extent that the term 'orphan drug' is often used to refer to those drugs for which the anticipated market is too small to (financially) justify a company undertaking the costly drug approval process (38). ICON6 again provides a telling example of the impact of regulations, and the system and resultant costs incurred in the evaluation process. The design of ICON6 had to be reconfigured part way through as the company behind the drug, AstraZeneca, decided to discontinue development after disappointing findings in clinical trials of its use for other types of cancer.

Together these three drivers have created the pressure, need, and space for innovation. A large literature exists on the statistical efficiency of various clinical trial designs to speed up the evaluation process by providing quicker results, or potentially providing more reliable results in terms of sequential assessments and studies. Alternative designs may also enable studies which require few participants. One related and corresponding aspect of sustained interest is the assessment of 'futility' in addition to 'efficacy', that is, stopping a clinical trial (and the evaluation process) early if a treatment does not seem likely to work based upon accumulating data. The issue of data monitoring in a clinical trial is considered in Chapter 7.

Clinical trials in other settings

Outside of the medicinal regulatory setting there is even greater variation in clinical trials. Clinical trials evaluating what is called 'off-label' use, that is, the use of a medicine for another purpose other than the one it was original approved for, are common (38). For example, azathioprine was originally approved for immune-response suppression in adults receiving transplant surgery but it is now regularly used for eczema with studies carried out to evaluate this 'off-label' use taking place later on (38). The growth of the evidence-based medicine movement in the latter part of the 20th century has led to the evidence underpinning all aspects of medical practice being questioned. Providing the best evidence to determine clinical care has become a key focus of modern medicine (39). Professional expectations of appropriate health professional practice have increased with the generation of detailed clinical guidance covering many common conditions in a number of countries. This guidance has also led in turn to a desire to generate research to support specific positions where the existing evidence is insufficient. Another important change has been the recognition of the need to produce summaries of all the available evidence on the treatment of conditions. This approach led to the founding of the Cochrane Collaboration in 1993 (retitled 'Cochrane' in 2015), named after Archie Cochrane, a pioneer who sought a scientific evidence base for medical practice, and who was an early advocate of RCTs. Cochrane's aim is to provide up-to-date reviews of evidence about the effects of healthcare. The natural lifecycle of clinically motivated research typically beginning with a systematic review of the current evidence. These reviews often identify the need for a new study to address a deficiency in the current evidence, and thus provide further academic stimulus for the initiation of new clinical trials. Governmental agencies (e.g. the National Institutes of Health (NIH) in the US, the National Institute for Health and Care Research (NIHR) in the UK, and Horizon Europe in the EU) and not-for-profit organizations and medical charities (e.g. the Cancer Research Institute in the US and the British Heart Foundation) began to take an increased role in the funding and commissioning of medical research over the last 30 years. They tended to focus on areas where commercial funding might need supplementing, or for which no commercial interest existed, thus providing the financial fuel to facilitate the conduct of research, including many clinical trials to address the increasingly apparent research needs. Greater focus on the patient perspective has also identified research questions to be addressed which had been previously neglected.

Clinical trials of non-drug treatments for clinical use

Clinical use of non-drug treatments, unless they are directly linked to a specific medical device, are not typically covered by legal requirements for evidence. For example, the ease with which a new surgical technique can be adopted into clinical practice has been noted as a source of serious concern. A clinical trial, typically an RCT, might only take place some time after a procedure has been used in routine clinical care. The widespread use of laparoscopic cholecystec-tomy, a substantially more difficult procedure for removing the gallbladder, without robust evaluation was a particularly infamous example in general surgery (40). A variety of frameworks for the evaluation of non-drug treatments have been proposed (41,42). These typically propose a place for clinical trials, and RCTs in particular (see Chapter 2) within them. Additionally, they have a general progression of exploratory or preliminary research through to a definitive evaluation. What is, and is not, a clinical trial in this context is not well defined. Reflecting on the definition provided at the beginning of this chapter, a great variety of studies which might be described as 'clinical trials' are possible. At a minimum, it should be a planned study on humans, carried out with a view to evaluate the safety and/or effect of a treatment or related care of some kind, and which involves data relating to a treatment's use and effect.

The pattern for non-drug treatments is roughly like that shown in Table 1.5, and is less elaborate than for clinical trials of drugs. Given the typical absence of regulatory approval, no phase 4 studies exist except in the sense of an evaluation after widespread clinical usage has occurred. Some initial small studies, followed by small RCTs, would typically occur prior to the conduct of a large (for the area) RCT. Phase 2 and 3/4 trials may or may not occur. The latter more definitive evaluations may ultimately be of a retrospective and observational nature, that is, not a clinical trial in the proper sense. An example phase 3 clinical trial of the simple addition of bath additives to treat eczema in children is described in Table 1.6 (see also Figure 1.5) (43).

Table 1.5 Clinical trials of non-drug treatments

Type	Phase 1	Phase 2	Phase 3/4
Main objective	Initial experience	Safety and efficacy	Safety and efficacy
Size	Circa 20–80	Circa 100–200	Circa 500
Population	Carefully selected patients (may be first in human)	Subset of clinical population thought to benefit	Clinical population receiving treatment
Design	Usually single arm, single centre	May be randomized, possibly multicentre	Randomized, multicentre
Control group	Unlikely	Maybe	Yes
Outcome	Surrogate/clinical	Surrogate/clinical often short term	Clinical/patient-focused short and longer term

Table 1.6 Phase 3 clinical trial—BATHE

Background	Childhood eczema is a common condition impacting quality of life. Clinical guidelines suggest using emollient to prevent flare-ups. Emollients can be given in different ways including by adding to bath water
Objective	To determine the clinical effectiveness and the cost-effectiveness of including emollient bath additives in the standard management of eczema in children
Design	Multicentre, phase 3 randomized controlled trial
Population	483 children aged 1–11 years (mean of 5 years) with atopic dermatitis in the UK
Treatments	One of two groups: • Intervention: prescribed emollient bath additives for 12 months of use in addition to standard care • Control: asked to not use bath additives for 12 months and only standard care
Study duration	49 months recruiting with median treatment and follow-up times of 8 and 20 months, respectively
Key findings	• 99% of the bath additives group versus only 13% of the no bath additives group used bath additives when they bathed • Average POEM score over 16-week period was 7.5 (SD 6.0) and 8.4 (SD 6.0) in the bath additives and no bath additives group • No statistical difference in the POEM was found between the groups over this period (Figure 1.5) • The groups did not differ in healthcare use, costs, or cost-effectiveness
Conclusions	• Addition of emollient bath additives to standard care did not improve quality of life
Registration	ISRCTN registry: ISRCTN84102309
Reference	Santer M, Ridd MJ, Francis NA, Stuart B, Rumsby K, Chorozoglou M, et al. Emollient bath additives for the treatment of childhood eczema (BATHE): multicentre pragmatic parallel group randomised controlled trial of clinical and cost effectiveness. BMJ. 2018;361:k1332

POEM, patient-orientated eczema measure; SD, standard deviation.

Other ways to describe clinical trials

A more recent and helpful distinction has been made between clinical trials which seek to assess 'efficacy', that is, whether a treatment works, versus 'effectiveness', that is whether a treatment works in the setting in which it will be used in clinical practice. The labels 'pragmatic' and 'explanatory' have been increasingly used to indicate the overarching focus on the study's evaluation. Alternatively, these studies might be described as (comparative) 'effectiveness' or 'efficacy' trials, respectively denoting overlapping but not exactly equivalent concepts. Furthermore, a distinction is often made between those studies

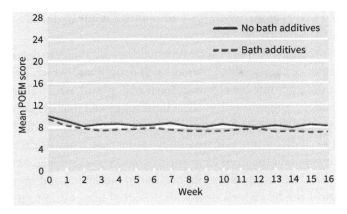

Figure 1.5 Patient-oriented eczema measure (POEM) scores during 16-week primary outcome period.

intended to provide a result from which action could be taken (e.g. phase 3 trials) and are 'definitive' studies, and those which are in essence designed to prepare for such a 'definitive' study (i.e. phase 0–2 clinical trials). Outside of the drug regulatory setting, terms such as pilot studies or trials, feasibility studies, and exploratory studies are commonly used to describe these preliminary/preparatory studies. Recognizing the difficulty of conducting a definitive clinical trial, even the feasibility of such a study, let alone its exact design and implementation, may be challenging (44). Accordingly, a feasibility study might be carried out to assess this.

Clinical trials in contemporary medicine

Over the last 100 years, clinical trials have grown greatly in number and spread throughout the world. The largest registry of clinical trials, ClinicalTrials.gov, has over 438,755 entries from 221 countries as of 16 January 2023. Of these, over 80,000 are purported to be still recruiting. Given this, it might seem odd to even consider the possibility of a world without clinical trials, or at least one in which the value of clinical trials is questioned. Nevertheless, some individuals have been critical of the conduct and value of clinical trials, and have questioned their role in medical evaluation. A variety of concerns, and alternative research approaches, have been proposed.

In the US, the desire to use a new drug as soon as it is ready has led to the 'right to try' a new drug under certain conditions even though it has not been approved for use (45). The onset of the coronavirus disease 2019 (COVID-19) pandemic led to lots of 'armchair epidemiologists' ready to declare a medicine as 'successful' from early reports.

Strong claims (some of them even rather wild) of the ability to determine with a high degree of certainty which patients will benefit and which will not from new treatments (e.g. some uses of 'machine learning' and 'artificial intelligence') have been made. More modestly, others have suggested that the advent of routine data systems has provided a much cheaper and quicker way to evaluate treatments (46). Furthermore, increasingly sophisticated statistical approaches can mimic or supplant the need for control patients (randomized or otherwise) under certain rather strong assumptions. Causal modelling and more complex epidemiological models which deal with potential biases due to unmeasured variables offer an attractive advance on simpler more traditional statistical modelling approaches. Their use could potentially reduce the need for clinical trials to some degree (at least when considering treatments which have previously undergone some safety assessment), or where safety is less of a concern. Lastly, in the context of the COVID-19 pandemic, some have questioned the value of the evidence-based medicine paradigm, particularly RCTs. Nevertheless, clinical trials are a fundamental part of the science of modern medicine and have been so for over 50 years. Remarkably, even after decades of research we are still understanding the benefits of a well-conducted clinical trial, and of a randomized comparison in particular (47,48). Even the recent COVID-19 pandemic, which is supposed by some to have exposed the weakness of clinical trials, has in fact shown that clinical trials, and RCTs in particular, can be conducted much quicker, and on a larger scale than even many of their strongest advocates dared to believe was still possible. Their use led to critical discoveries in the treatment (49) and the vaccination of people (50) from this disease while understanding of the virus and its transmission was still embryonic. Thus, it seems safe to think that clinical trials will be used for many years to come. Their design will no doubt undergo some further evolution. However, for the foreseeable future and beyond, clinical trials are here to stay, helping us identify improvements in medical care, and improving the health of humanity.

The rest of the book

Chapter 2 considers the basic components of a standard clinical trial, and how it should be designed. Following this, Chapter 3 discusses in some depth the RCT design as the optimal clinical trial design. Chapter 4 covers alternative RCT designs which could be used. Chapter 5 examines the question of how many individuals need to be included in clinical trials, followed by how a clinical trial can be set-up (Chapter 6), and how data should be collected and monitored (Chapter 7). Chapter 8 considers how to actually conduct a clinical trial, followed by how it should be analysed (Chapter 9), and finally how to report the findings of the clinical trial (Chapter 10).

References

1. Lind J. A treatise of the scurvy. In three parts. Containing an inquiry into the nature, causes and cure, of that disease. Together with a critical and chronological view of what has been published on the subject. Edinburgh: Sands, Murray and Cochran for A Kincaid and A Donaldson; 1753.
2. Donovan J, Mills N, Smith M, Brindle L, Jacoby A, Peters T, et al. Quality improvement report: improving design and conduct of randomised trials by embedding them in qualitative research: ProtecT (prostate testing for cancer and treatment) study. Commentary: presenting unbiased information to patients can be difficult. BMJ. 2002;325(7367):766–70.
3. Sinha G. United Kingdom becomes the cancer clinical trials recruitment capital of the world. Journal of the National Cancer Institute. 2007;99(6):420–2.
4. Tröhler U. James Lind and the evaluation of clinical practice. The James Lind Library. 2003. Available from: https://www.jameslindlibrary.org/articles/james-lind-and-the-evaluation-of-clinical-practice/
5. Meldrum ML. A brief history of the randomized controlled trial. From oranges and lemons to the gold standard. Hematology/Oncology Clinics of North America. 2000;14(4):745–60, vii.
6. Chalmers I, Dukan E, Podolsky SH, Davey Smith G. The advent of fair treatment allocation schedules in clinical trials during the 19th and early 20th centuries. Journal of the Royal Society of Medicine. 2012;105(5):221–7.
7. The James Lind Library. 1.2 Why treatment comparisons are essential. The James Lind Library. n.d. Available from: https://www.jameslindlibrary.org/essays/1-2-why-treatment-comparisons-are-essential/
8. The James Lind Library. 2.2 The need to compare like-with-like in treatment comparisons. The James Lind Library. n.d. Available from: https://www.jameslindlibrary.org/essays/2-2-the-need-to-compare-like-with-like-in-treatment-comparisons/
9. Chalmers I. Assembling comparison groups to assess the effects of health care. Journal of the Royal Society of Medicine. 1997;90(7):379–86.
10. Hill AB. The clinical trial. New England Journal of Medicine. 1952;247:113–19.
11. Lilienfeld AM. The Fielding H. Garrison Lecture. Ceteris paribus: the evolution of the clinical trial. Bulletin of the History of Medicine. 1982;56(1):1–18.
12. Doll R. Controlled trials: the 1948 watershed. BMJ. 1998;317(7167):1217–20.
13. Armitage P. Fisher, Bradford Hill, and randomization. International Journal of Epidemiology. 2003;32(6):925–8.
14. A Special Committee of the Medical Research Council. Clinical trials of antihistaminic drugs in the prevention and treatment of the common cold; report by a special committee of the Medical Research Council. British Medical Journal. 1950;2(4676):425–9.
15. Cook JA. The challenges faced in the design, conduct and analysis of surgical randomised controlled trials. Trials. 2009;10:9.
16. Dawson L. The Salk Polio Vaccine Trial of 1954: risks, randomization and public involvement in research. Clinical Trials. 2004;1(1):122–30.

17. Bothwell LE, Greene JA, Podolsky SH, Jones DS. Assessing the gold standard—lessons from the history of RCTs. New England Journal of Medicine. 2016;374(22):2175–81.

18. Cassidy A. 'Big science' in the field: experimenting with badgers and bovine TB, 1995–2015. History and Philosophy of the Life Sciences. 2015;37(3):305–25.

19. Doll R. Clinical trials: retrospect and prospect. Statistics in Medicine. 1982;1(4):337–44.

20. Tantibanchachai C. US regulatory response to thalidomide (1950–2000). The Embryo Project Encyclopedia. 1 April 2014. Available from: embryo.asu.edu/pages/us-regulatory-response-thalidomide-1950-2000

21. Weijer C, Enkin MW, Shapiro SH, Glass KC. Clinical equipoise and not the uncertainty principle is the moral underpinning of the randomised controlled trial—for & against. BMJ. 2000;321(7263):756.

22. Wikipedia contributors. Unethical human experimentation. Wikipedia, The Free Encyclopedia. 30 August 2020. Available from: https://en.wikipedia.org/wiki/Unethical_human_experimentation

23. Weyzig F, Schipper I. #1: examples of unethical trials. SOMO briefing paper on ethics in clinical trials. The Centre for Research on Multinational Corporations (SOMO). 2008. Available from: https://www.somo.nl/wp-content/uploads/2008/02/Examples-of-unethical-trials.pdf

24. Senn S, Amin D, Bailey RA, Bird SM, Bogacka B, Colman P, et al. Statistical issues in first-in-man studies. Journal of the Royal Statistical Society Series A. 2007;170(3):517–79.

25. International Council for Harmonisation of Technical Requirements for Pharmaceuticals for Human Use (ICH). Efficacy guidelines. Available from: https://www.ich.org/page/efficacy-guidelines

26. Illingworth Research Group. GCP—important changes through time. Illingworth Research Group. 2020. Available from: https://illingworthresearch.com/good-clinical-practice-a-brief-history/

27. Vijayananthan A, Nawawi O. The importance of good clinical practice guidelines and its role in clinical trials. Biomedical Imaging and Intervention Journal. 2008;4(1):e5.

28. Schipper I. Clinical Trials in Developing Countries: How to Protect People Against Unethical Practices? Brussels: Directorate-General for External Policies of the Union, European Parliament; 2009.

29. Eisenhauer EA, Twelves C, Buyse M. Phase I Cancer Clinical Trials: A Practical Guide. 2nd ed. New York: Oxford University Press; 2015.

30. National Cancer Institute. Maximum tolerated dose. National Cancer Institute. n.d. Available from: https://www.cancer.gov/publications/dictionaries/cancer-terms/def/maximum-tolerated-dose

31. Schenk DB, Koller M, Ness DK, Griffith SG, Grundman M, Zago W, et al. First-in-human assessment of PRX002, an anti-α-synuclein monoclonal antibody, in healthy volunteers. Movement Disorders. 2017;32(2):211–18.

32. Jankovic J, Goodman I, Safirstein B, Marmon TK, Schenk DB, Koller M, et al. Safety and tolerability of multiple ascending doses of PRX002/RG7935, an anti-α-synuclein monoclonal antibody, in patients with Parkinson disease: a randomized clinical trial. JAMA Neurology. 2018;75(10):1206–14.

33. Pagano G, Taylor KI, Anzures-Cabrera J, Marchesi M, Simuni T, Marek K, et al. Trial of prasinezumab in early-stage Parkinson's disease. New England Journal of Medicine. 2022;387(5):421–32.

34. Ledermann JA, Embleton AC, Raja F, Perren TJ, Jayson GC, Rustin GJS, et al. Cediranib in patients with relapsed platinum-sensitive ovarian cancer (ICON6): a randomised, double-blind, placebo-controlled phase 3 trial. Lancet. 2016;387(10023):1066–74.

35. The Council of the European Economic Community. Council directive of 26 January 1965 on the approximation of provisions laid down by law, regulation or administrative action relating to proprietary medicinal products. Official Journal of the European Communities. 1965;22:369–73.

36. Collier R. Drug development cost estimates hard to swallow. CMAJ: Canadian Medical Association Journal. 2009;180(3):279–80.
37. Kearns P. The need for proportionate regulation of clinical trials. Lancet Oncology. 2013;14(6):454–5.
38. Wittich CM, Burkle CM, Lanier WL. Ten common questions (and their answers) about off-label drug use. Mayo Clinic Proceedings. 2012;87(10):982–90.
39. Masic I, Miokovic M, Muhamedagic B. Evidence based medicine—new approaches and challenges. Acta Informatica Medica. 2008;16(4):219–25.
40. Meakins JL. Innovation in surgery: the rules of evidence. American Journal of Surgery. 2002;183(4):399–405.
41. McCulloch P, Altman DG, Campbell WB, Flum DR, Glasziou P, Marshall JC, et al. No surgical innovation without evaluation: the IDEAL recommendations. Lancet. 2009;374(9695):1105–12.
42. Craig P, Dieppe P, Macintyre S, Michie S, Nazareth I, Petticrew M. Developing and evaluating complex interventions: the new Medical Research Council guidance. BMJ. 2008;337:a1655.
43. Santer M, Ridd MJ, Francis NA, Stuart B, Rumsby K, Chorozoglou M, et al. Emollient bath additives for the treatment of childhood eczema (BATHE): multicentre pragmatic parallel group randomised controlled trial of clinical and cost effectiveness. BMJ. 2018;361:k1332.
44. Eldridge SM, Chan CL, Campbell MJ, Bond CM, Hopewell S, Thabane L, et al. CONSORT 2010 statement: extension to randomised pilot and feasibility trials. BMJ. 2016;355:i5239.
45. US Food and Drug Administration. Right to try. Food and Drug Administration. 2020 (updated 13 September 2022). Available from: https://www.fda.gov/patients/learn-about-expanded-access-and-other-treatment-options/right-try
46. Caliebe A, Leverkus F, Antes G, Krawczak M. Does big data require a methodological change in medical research? BMC Medical Research Methodology. 2019;19(1):125.
47. Labrecque JA, Swanson SA. Target trial emulation: teaching epidemiology and beyond. European Journal of Epidemiology. 2017;32(6):473–5.
48. Bellamy SL, Lin JY, Ten Have TR. An introduction to causal modeling in clinical trials. Clinical Trials. 2007;4(1):58–73.
49. Nuffield Department of Population Health. RECOVERY trial. University of Oxford. n.d. Available from: https://www.recoverytrial.net/
50. Knoll MD, Wonodi C. Oxford-AstraZeneca COVID-19 vaccine efficacy. Lancet. 2021;397(10269):72–4.

2
Designing a clinical trial

> The design of every clinical trial starts with a primary clinical research question.
>
> **Scott Evans, 2010 (1)**

Where to start

Clinical trial design involves a number of key decisions related to various methodological and practice aspects in order to come to an implementable design. The basic study design, definitions of the treatments, sample size, and statistical analysis might well be the first things that spring to mind. However, we begin with the most foundational aspect of any study design: the research question which the study is intended to answer.

Defining the main research question

At first glance, the reason for conducting a clinical trial might seem so obvious that spending time refining and clarifying it might seem unnecessary. Questions such as does the new Parkinson's drug work, what is the right dose of this drug to give patients with hypertension, and should these patients (should I) have surgery or physiotherapy for their (my) anterior cruciate ligament injury readily come up in clinical practice and medical care. They are simple and intuitive, and motivate the need for, and the idea of generating, new research including a clinical trial. In reality, such simple research questions are not directly implementable and can be addressed (in designing and conducting a clinical trial) in a surprisingly great variety of ways. Getting the main research question right is of critical importance for undertaking an informative clinical trial. A poor research question can lead to a study which cannot be completed, or cannot be conducted well. It can also lead to unnecessary confusion and make the process of designing the study more difficult than necessary. Furthermore, even if all goes to plan in terms of conducting the trial, it may end up being one which has limited value and impact.

This can be because it addresses a question that no one is overly interested in. Or it is a study which few can apply the findings of. Clearly articulating what we wish to address helps if, and when, we are required to make strategic decisions later on due to unexpected occurrences. Rather surprisingly, the research question is not always clearly expressed even in the journal article reporting a study's findings (2,3). There is reason to expect, and some empirical evidence to support the belief, that studies with better formulated research questions tend to have better methods and also a better standard of reporting once published (3). Additionally, there is reason to think that these studies will be more influential. A useful overview of relevant resources is provided elsewhere (4).

Focusing on and confirming the main research question to be answered is of critical importance, and a key step in designing a clinical trial (4). As clinical trials are very expensive to conduct and often present unique opportunities to collect additional data, increasingly clinical trials often seek to address multiple research questions. However, one needs to know which research question takes primacy, as all research studies involve decisions and prioritization of resources, and which research questions and aspects are of secondary, or ancillary, concern. Various approaches have been used to articulate what the proposed research study is trying to achieve and to express this. A useful approach is to be able to articulate a single overarching research question which the study will seek to address. The response to the research question can be expressed as a primary objective of the research study. Some studies might have two if they complement each other. Beyond this there may be multiple secondary objectives which are supportive of, or are ancillary, to the primary objective. For example, for a phase 3 trial comparing two knee surgery (total and partial knee replacement) operations for the treatment of inner (medial) knee osteoarthritis, the main research question could be whether there is a difference in the knee-related quality of life (e.g. pain and function) between the two operations. The corresponding study primary objective would then be 'to assess the knee-related quality of life' after these operations 'for patients with medial knee osteoarthritis'. However, there are various ways we could then assess 'knee-related quality of life' which could lead to slightly different objectives. Nevertheless, one of these needs to be selected to be the primary objective which in turn should be reflected in the choice of the primary outcome. The primary outcome is the main outcome from which the main result of the study is to be determined. Similarly, we could also look at safety though this might not be the primary objective of the study, but it could be a natural secondary objective.

Developing the outline of the research design

We will now consider how to flesh out our crude initial research idea into a well-defined research question. Our initial question can be put more specifically: do the two operations differ in terms of knee-related pain and function in treating knee osteoarthritis? The simplicity of the question hides the context and without fleshing this out it is clearly not one we could implement. This question prompts many other related questions—how should the operations be performed, when, and by whom? For whom and how will we measure 'knee-related pain and function'? Who are we trying to provide evidence for with this study? A helpful framework to consider how we might go about developing the initial crude research question we have is called *PICOTS*; this acronym stands for Population, Intervention, Control (sometimes described as a 'comparator'), Outcome, Timing, and Setting (Table 2.1). A well-defined research question is one for which we have a clear definition for each of these core components.

For each of the six components there are various potential options and some of the more common options are shown in Table 2.1. For the population aspect of the research question, it might seem obvious that these are patients of some kind. However, this is not necessarily the case. As we saw in Chapter 1, some early phase trials use healthy volunteers. If we are evaluating a vaccine, not only are the intended participant not patients but they could be anyone. Even if we are interested in the treatment of patients there are different options, such as those newly diagnosed, persistent disease, recurrence, or varying severities of disease. Furthermore, a distinction can be made between the initial treatment of these patient groups and ongoing treatment for disease of a more chronic nature (e.g. irritable bowel disease). Example responses are also given in Table 2.1 for a clinical trial seeking to evaluate the use of chemotherapy alongside surgery for the treatment of bowel cancer.

Clinical trial examples

We now consider in turn two examples in more depth to see how the initial idea might be developed into a research question and then into the objectives which frame the clinical trial design. The first example involves designing a clinical trial for a new drug for Parkinson's disease. The second relates to surgery for medial knee osteoarthritis, as considered earlier in this chapter.

Table 2.1 PICOTS framework with common options and bowel cancer example

Element	Description	Common options	Bowel cancer example
Population	The individuals who will take part in the study	• Members of the public • Healthy volunteers • Individuals at risk of a disease • Newly diagnosed individuals • Individuals with persistent disease (i.e. have been treated before unsuccessfully) • Individuals with recurrence disease (disease which was in remission but has returned) • Individuals with advanced/severe disease	Newly diagnosed patients with bowel cancer
Intervention(s)	How will the intervention(s) to be evaluated be given?	• Drug tablet • Intravenous drug • Radiotherapy • Surgery • Educational material • Psychotherapy • Exercise • Dietary guidance	Course of chemotherapy before and after surgical excision of the tumour
Control	What, if any, alternative will there be to which the intervention treatment can be directly compared?	• No control • No additional action • Placebo • Competitor treatment	Standard care which consists of chemotherapy using standard agent after surgical excision of the tumour
Outcome(s)	What will be the primary way of assessing whether the intervention treatment has an effect or not?	• Occurrence of disease • Progression of disease • Intervention-related adverse events (e.g. toxicity) • Death • Patient-reported outcome (e.g. assessment of symptoms or disease-severity) • Laboratory-assessed biomarker (e.g. cholesterol level) • Imaging-based outcome (e.g. healing of fracture based upon computed tomography scan)	Progression of disease or death

Table 2.1 Continued

Element	Description	Common options	Bowel cancer example
Timing	Over what timescale will individuals be involved in the study?	• 24 hours • 7 days • 30 days • 90 days • 6 months • 1 year • 5 years	Average of 2 years of follow-up
Setting	Where will the study be conducted?	• Research facility • Family doctor practice • Pharmacy • Local hospital • Teaching (university hospital) • Local community	Routine medical care hospital setting

Parkinson's drug example

For an early phase clinical trial of a drug for Parkinson's disease we might articulate our initial queries as something like the following: is the drug safe to use, and what dose should be given? The relationships between the initial queries, the research question, and the objectives which structure the clinical trial design are illustrated in Figure 2.1. The initial queries or uncertainties need to be addressed before we can move on and think about the optimal dose, and quantifying the treatment effects (whether they be positive or negative) in a suitable clinical setting. To have a researchable question we need to be more specific about what we are interested in. Commonly in drug development PK is considered separately from PD though both are clearly crucial considerations in ultimately deciding upon a suitable dose, and of the safety of the drug more generally. We may decide, as in the study we saw in Chapter 1, that we wish to consider the effects in health participants given how little we currently know about the drug. Furthermore, we might decide we want to prioritize knowledge about the PK at this point. Our main (primary) outcome measure, so as to match our interest in the PK of the drug, could be the serum PRX002 concentration. Progressing with this primary objective of assessing PD we can flesh this out towards an implementable research study using the PICOTS framework. A focus on healthy individuals would be a reasonable choice at a very early point of understanding of a new drug. We can define how we will deliver the intervention and whether we have a control or not. In this

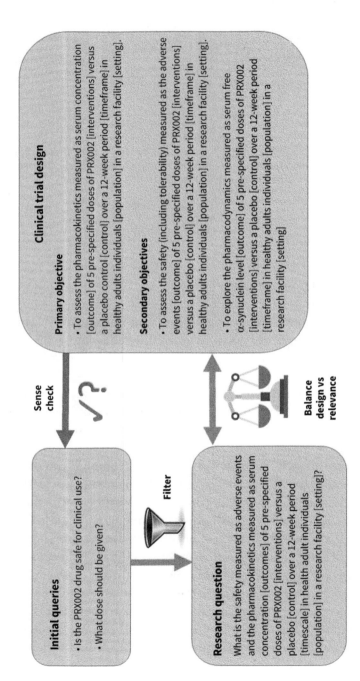

Figure 2.1 PRX002 for Parkinson's disease example—research question and study objectives.

Clinical trial design

Primary objective

• To assess the pharmacokinetics measured as serum concentration [outcome] of 5 pre-specified doses of PRX002 [interventions] versus a placebo control [control] over a 12-week period [timeframe] in healthy adults individuals [population] in a research facility [setting].

Secondary objectives

• To assess the safety (including tolerability) measured as the adverse events [outcome] of 5 pre-specified doses of PRX002 [interventions] versus a placebo [control] over a 12-week period [timeframe] in healthy adults individuals [population] in a research facility [setting].

• To explore the pharmacodynamics measured as serum free α-synuclein level [outcome] of 5 pre-specified doses of PRX002 [interventions] versus a placebo [control] over a 12-week period [timeframe] in healthy adults individuals [population] in a research facility [setting]

Sense check

Balance design vs relevance

Initial queries

• Is the PRX002 drug safe for clinical use?

• What dose should be given?

Filter

Research question

What is the safety measured as adverse events and the pharmacokinetics measured as serum concentration [outcomes] of 5 pre-specified doses of PRX002 [interventions] versus a placebo [control] over a 12-week period [timescale] in health adult individuals [population] in a research facility [setting]?

case, choosing an intravenous injection of one of five doses or a normal saline (placebo control) as was done in the Schenk et al. study we saw in Chapter 1 seems like a reasonable option (5). This would help inform the dose choice in subsequent studies. For timescale we could opt for 12 weeks of follow-up with more frequent early measurements in the first 24 hours than later in the follow-up period (e.g. also assessing at 1 and 3 days and then at 1, 2, 4, 6, and 12 weeks after infusion). Lastly, we might plan to conduct the clinical trial within a single centre with suitable facilities for the required intensive monitoring needed, particularly in the first 8 hours. It is worth noting that each of these clarifications makes the question our study is going to answer more specific. This has implications for its practicality in delivery, and its applicability in terms of to whom and when the results apply.

Therefore, we might articulate the main research question as *what is the PK measured as serum concentration [outcome] of five pre-specified doses of PRX002 [interventions] versus a placebo [control] over a 12-week period [time frame] in healthy adult individuals [population] in a research facility [setting]?* Correspondingly, our study's primary objective could be *to assess the PK measured as the serum concentration [outcome] of five pre-specified doses of PRX002 [interventions] versus a placebo control [control] over a 12-week period [time frame] in healthy adult individuals [population] in a research facility [setting].*

Having confirmed the main research question we are seeking to ask and the corresponding primary objective of the study we hope to address, it is natural to go on to consider if we can also address other relevant queries. As long as it does not compromise addressing the primary objective, this will add value to the study. We could address our other query related to safety by including a secondary objective to assess the safety (including tolerability) measured as *the occurrence of adverse events [outcome] with five pre-specified doses of PRX002 [interventions] versus a placebo control [control] over a 12-week period [time frame] in healthy adult individuals [population] in a research facility [setting].* In a similar manner, we might also wish to assess the PD of PRX002 in healthy participants and to correspondingly include a further secondary objective to address this. Collecting data on PD is readily done alongside safety and PK data. It is also a natural accompaniment and indeed was an objective of the Schenk et al. study (5) we saw in Chapter 1. It is worth noting there is a choice here, and one that needs to be carefully considered in light of what is already known. It is not necessary for PK to be the focus of the primary objective in our study. It could have been safety assessed as occurrence of adverse events or something else. Alternatively, if there was already a good understanding of the PK properties of the drug, perhaps as it had been used for other conditions, the main focus reflected in the research question might have been on PD. Or alternatively, it could have been both PD and PK together to characterize the relationship between these aspects of the drug properties. This can be approached from a modelling perspective to varying degrees of complexity, which in turn lead to specific data requirements, and practical study implications. Once we have chosen our primary and secondary objectives, we can make a sense check of the proposed objectives against the initial queries to make sure we have not deviated too far away from our original concerns. In this case all seems straightforward and reasonable. In passing we note that the design of a study can change substantially (and not always to everyone's realization) when multiple people input into the development of the study concept over multiple occasions. Therefore, regularly referring back to the original concepts is a key part of good practice in clinical trial design. Figure 2.1 shows the basic process of formulating the main research question and objectives of the clinical trial for the PRX002 example.

Knee replacement example

We now consider a second clinical trial example based upon the Total or Partial Knee Arthroplasty Trial (TOPKAT) RCT (6). The relationships between the initial query, the research question, and the objectives which structure the clinical trial design are shown in Figure 2.2. Patients with severe knee osteoarthritis require surgery to replace the knee joint to relieve pain and improve mobility. Two types of implants are available when only the inner part of the (medial) knee is affected. A total replacement of the whole of the knee joint or a partial replacement of only the diseased (inner) area can be carried out. Both operations are in clinical use though the partial knee operation leads to a more complicated operation and is less commonly conducted. Patients seek treatment to deal with pain, stiffness, and restricted function accompanying the disease. Each operation may have its own, though similar, pattern of complications. It may affect the overall health-related quality of life differently. There may be different needs for further treatments and cost implications. It is unclear which of the two options should be the preferred operation from the patient's perspective. It would be natural therefore to conduct a clinical trial to compare these two operations. We might formulate the research question as follows: *is there a difference in the knee-related quality of life between total and partial knee replacement for patients with osteoarthritis of the medial knee within the UK National Health Service (NHS)?*

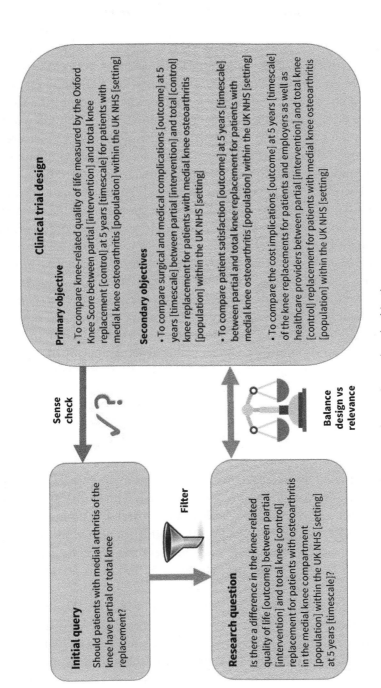

Figure 2.2 Knee arthritis surgery example—research question and study objectives.

Various measures have been used to assess patient-reported quality of life for knee conditions; a commonly used one, developed for this setting, is the Oxford Knee Score (OKS) (7). This score was specifically designed and developed to assess function and pain after total knee replacement from the patient's perspective. Many surgeons view 5 years as the first key time point for assessing the outcome of the operations. It is seen as when failure of the surgery has started to occur more commonly, and a point when the recovery pathway for the operation becomes clearer. Lastly, the operation could be delivered in various settings. We could seek to assess the outcome following treatment in private hospitals; however, the overwhelming majority of operations of this kind in the UK are conducted within the NHS. As experience of the operation is required, we might pre-specify our criteria for surgeons to have some prior experience of both operations. Putting this all together, our study's primary objective might therefore be *to assess whether there is a difference at 5 years [time frame] in the knee-related quality of life measured primarily by the OKS [outcome] between partial [intervention] and total knee replacement [control] for patients with medial knee osteoarthritis [population] delivered within the UK NHS system [setting] by experienced surgeons.* We can then add secondary objectives to address our other related queries which would inform the choice of operations. Corresponding secondary objectives can be added looking at medical and surgical complications, patient satisfaction, and the cost implications of the operations.

Is my research question a good one to address?

The above discussion is related to defining the main research question. However, a well-defined question is not necessarily a good one to seek to address. A helpful way to evaluate whether our research question is a sensible one is the FINER criteria (8) (Table 2.2). FINER stands for feasible, interesting, novel, ethical, and relevant. Each of these five domains is fairly self-explanatory but is briefly summarized here:

1. First, we should ask whether the research question we have opted for is one that we think is *feasible* to address; can it be answered in a study that we can imagine being conducted? Are there likely to be enough potential participants? Can the intervention and control, if there is one, be delivered in the way needed? Do we have a way to assess the outcome we are most interested in? Could it realistically be conducted quickly enough in a reasonable number of centres without costing too much? Assessing

Table 2.2 FINER criteria

Domain	Questions to ask
Feasible	• Will there be enough potential participants for the study? • Can the intervention (and control) be delivered as needed? • Can the outcome be measured as needed? • Are there suitable centres to conduct the study in? • How long might the study take? • Are sufficient funds available?
Interesting	• Is it an exciting question to ask? • Will key stakeholders take notice of the findings? • Would anyone fund the study as they want to know the answer?
Novel	• Has the question been fully answered before? • How will this study differ from previous studies?
Ethical	• Would I be willing to take part if I was eligible? • Would my colleagues consider it appropriate to conduct? • What kind of risk will individuals taking part be exposed to?
Relevant	• Does it have the potential to alter clinical practice (or will it lead to a study that could do so)? • Will healthcare decision-makers be influenced by the findings? • Will patients be more informed given the findings? • Does it meet professional and regulatory body expectations?

feasibility will typically not be answered simply as a yes or no. Indeed, a full research study (feasibility study) of its own might be conducted to help us come to a conclusion on that matter. Nevertheless, considering this at an early stage of trial design is prudent.

2. The next question to ask oneself is if it is an *interesting* research question. Life is too short, and clinical trials are too demanding, expensive, and time-consuming to focus upon topics of little importance. So, have we articulated a question that excites anyone (including oneself!)? Will stakeholders take note of it? Is it one that someone would be prepared to fund to see it conducted?

3. Is it *novel*, are we planning something that is new that adds to what has already been done and new? This is not always as clear as it might appear as novelty can be subtle. However, we do not want to conduct a study to address a research question which has been well answered by many studies before. For example, our proposed study may not be the only one to compare the intervention and control treatments of interest to us but perhaps the population is different from previous studies. Or previous studies have not been conducted on a sufficient scale, and in a rigorous enough manner.

4. Next, we must consider if it is an *ethical* study to conduct? Is it one that someone independent from us would consider appropriate to conduct?

Will it be acceptable to stakeholders (especially patients and health professionals)? If you (or a loved one) were eligible, would you be willing to take part, or be happy for them to take part? Different people may view things somewhat differently in this regard, but if we do not ask ourselves the question, we may find ourselves in difficulty later. There will be various stages in developing a research idea where this can be assessed and we will get feedback from others (internal institutional reviews, funding proposal assessments, and regulatory approvals processes including ethical review). A key barometer is the views of those who will help deliver the study as well as those who we wish to participate in it. At this point we need to do an initial ethical sense check and sharing the outline proposal with colleagues is a good place to start.

5. Last, would it be a *relevant* question to answer? It might surprise some to know that a good study might be conducted which is interesting, novel, and ethical and yet it has little practical relevance. Nevertheless, that can be the case, if it represents too artificial a scenario. This is perhaps more pertinent for studies conducted outside of a regulatory drug setting. Such studies ultimately seek to directly influence clinical and patient practice, and healthcare systems. For example, a drug may have been given in our clinical trial daily by infusion for 7 days over 3-hour periods. However, the relevant clinical application might require it to be given as a single large ('bolus') infusion. As a consequence, the transferability of the findings from the trial would naturally be questioned even if the patient population and other aspects seem relevant. Furthermore, we may ask, does the study provide the information that patients need to make an informed choice about their treatment? Similarly, will healthcare professionals and decision-makers take note of the findings—does it address their needs and concerns?

Outline of a clinical trial

Having worked out our research question in some detail and the objectives of our study, we now need to move on to fleshing out our proposal. There is, or at least ought to be, therefore, a strong link between the research question posed, the objectives of the study, and the study which is designed. It is worth noting at the outset that designing a clinical trial (including the formulation of the research question) is not a sequential process but more like carving a sculpture—always viewing each decision and action in light of the overall vision (research question) to avoid going awry. An outline of the basic structure of a clinical trial is given in Figure 2.3.

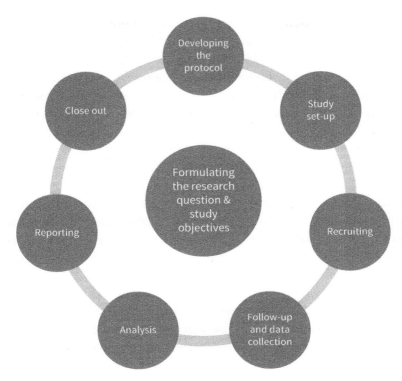

Figure 2.3 Outline of a clinical trial.

As with all good research studies, the first step in delivering a clinical trial begins with finalizing the study processes and documenting them so that they can be assessed and implemented, and that there is a record of what was intended. An initial idea needs to be refined and expanded upon. Once it has been fleshed out to an appropriate level, funding and approvals can be sought. In order to conduct the study, we need to set out what will happen in sufficient detail. A document called a protocol should be used to describe the study and all the related processes and steps in sufficient detail so that someone with no prior knowledge of the study would know what it entails, and to clarify the implementation of the study in practice. The protocol serves a number of different and important purposes. It should state in sufficient detail the implications for participants and others who would be involved in its running so that this can be assessed. Furthermore, it should state clearly what the study is intended to achieve, that is, the research question(s) it will seek to answer, and the objectives which are intended to be addressed. An explanation of why the study is being conducted and how it addresses this should be provided.

In set-up, the related documents and systems required to conduct the study need to be prepared along with any final approvals being secured. Typically this would involve an ethical assessment of the study by people not involved in this study. Once this has been received and all systems and personnel are in place and initiated into the study, recruitment can begin. Recruitment continues to the intended sample size (see Chapter 5 for consideration of how this number is determined) unless the study is stopped early. Data collection takes places immediately from the start of the recruitment process (see Chapters 6–8). Once data is available, the analysis of this data can take place (see Chapter 9). Once complete, this will be reported to others (most notably, in one or more research publications, but by no means is this the only way—see Chapter 10). To complete the clinical trial, a process of closure takes place where all documentation is stored in case it is needed in the future, and increasingly data is prepared for making it available to other interested individuals (usually research groups). While the above may give the impression of sequential tasks, the reality is that once a clinical trial completes set-up, the other steps of recruitment, follow-up and data collection, analysis, and reporting can take place at various overlapping periods until it is time for the final step of study closure. This book seeks to provide an introduction to these steps. We now consider some key decisions in trial design related to the specification of the study objectives.

Key decisions in formulating the study objectives

Superiority, equivalence, and inferiority statistical framing

Implicitly, the objectives of a typical phase 3 clinical trial are typically formulated as what is known statistically as a superiority question. This is to answer the question of whether there is a difference, that is, is one treatment superior to the other? It might be stated, as we have done earlier in this chapter, as 'to compare treatments X and Y' (i.e. to decide if there is a difference or not). There are, however, other ways to formulate the question into something which can be statistically assessed. The most common alternatives are equivalence and non-inferiority questions which should be reflected in the design of the respective clinical trial. In some settings we might not anticipate, or necessarily need a benefit, beyond the conventional treatment. We may merely wish to show a new treatment is not worse (i.e. 'non-inferior'). If we wanted to show that two treatments had the same level of effect, we could seek to show they are 'equivalent'. For example, if we consider the knee surgery example previously discussed, we might define our objective as to assess whether the knee-related quality of life of these two operations for a patient with medial osteoarthritis of the knee are equivalent. Clearly, we would need to decide what we mean by 'equivalent'. Alternatively, we could perhaps only want to show that partial knee replacement is 'non-inferior' to (i.e. not worse than) total knee replacement. In this case we might write out our research question as 'to assess whether partial knee replacement is non-inferior to total knee replacement in terms of the knee-related quality of life of these two operations for patient with medial osteoarthritis of the knee'. Why might we frame our question in this way? We may think that partial knee replacement had a clear benefit in some aspect (e.g. a key outcome, cost, or perhaps (though not in this case) ease of conduct). Given such a scenario, we might then only be concerned with showing it was 'non-inferior'. However, partial knee replacement was thought by some to be potentially better in some outcomes and worse for others. Therefore an 'equivalence' trial would have been a more appropriate choice than a 'non-inferiority' one had a 'superiority' framing not been used. The TOPKAT trial was designed to address a superiority question (allowing for total or partial knee replacement to be superior for different outcomes) (6). Accordingly, the primary objective was 'to assess the clinical effectiveness and cost-effectiveness of total knee replacement compared with partial (unicompartmental) knee replacement in patients with medial compartment osteoarthritis of the knee'. While the word 'superiority' is not used, the word 'compared' implies the same (i.e. either operation being superior, and any magnitude is of interest hence not looking at equivalence or non-inferiority). The terms 'clinical' and 'cost' before effectiveness clarify the general ways in which effectiveness will be assessed (both purely based upon clinical outcomes ('clinical effectiveness') and also via health economic evaluation ('cost-effectiveness')). The term 'effectiveness' implies multiple assessments, though as per our examples above there is arguably value in having more specific objectives which detail each aspect of the outcomes that are of interest.

Pragmatic and explanatory trials

As we saw earlier, the PICOTS framework can be helpful to clarify the outline of the research study in response to our research question. It is important to think through the coherence of the elements that are combined together as we develop our clinical trial design. One helpful way to think about this is to consider what is a 'pragmatic' as opposed to an 'explanatory' research question and the corresponding impact upon the study design. A pragmatic trial can be defined as one which is seeking to directly inform healthcare or policy decision-making and therefore is focused on the effect of the treatment in a typical clinical setting. In contrast, we may be interested in whether the treatment works in what we might consider to be an optimal (or at least favourable) setting, that is, an explanatory approach. We can take pretty much any research question and modify it accordingly to suit either approach and develop our study design using the PICOTS framework. It is worth noting that the explanatory approach matches up well with the concept of 'efficacy', and the approach typically adopted in the regulatory pharmaceutical setting, whereas a pragmatic focus is more associated with the concept of clinical 'effectiveness' and day-to-day clinical care questions.

In reality, there is no strict dichotomy of pragmatic and explanatory clinical trials but a variety of different options for different aspects of the study design. The PRECIS-2 (PRagmatic Explanatory Continuum Indicator Summary-2) tool (9) has been proposed to help with the design of RCTs and to help researchers think through how pragmatic or not the study design is (Table 2.3). It uses a five-point scale (ranging from 'very explanatory' to 'very pragmatic') for nine different domains (or aspects) of the study design ranging from eligibility criteria and recruitment through follow-up, primary outcome, and analysis approach. While designed explicitly for RCTs, the general approach has value for all clinical trials. By assessing the options for each of the domains it helps us think through the choices we are often implicitly making and how they map back to our original research question.

The choice of control

The decision regarding the control treatment is another of the key steps in defining the study's research question and study design. There are strong scientific reasons for desiring to include a control group in studies as we have seen in Chapter 1. We will consider this further in Chapter 3. A variety of potential options are available but broadly speaking as we progress from early phase 0/1 through to phase 4, studies are more likely to have a control. Furthermore, the control is more likely to represent the clinical alternative that a patient might be offered. Typically phase 0 or 1 trials do not have a control group, whereas phase 2 and 3 trials do. For trials conducted outside of the regulatory setting (See Chapter 6), there are often multiple options for potential comparators which could be selected as the control treatment. Often there is an existing treatment, or alternative new treatments. The more the treatments differ, the greater the contrast between the treatments being evaluated in the trial.

Table 2.3 Different ways to think about the research question

Statistical

Question type	Question form	Example
Superiority	Is there a difference between the treatment and control?	To assess whether partial knee replacement or total knee replacement is superior in terms of the knee-related quality of life as measured using the Oxford Knee Score after these two operations for patients with medial compartment osteoarthritis of the knee
Equivalence	Are the treatment and control equivalent?	To assess whether partial knee replacement is equivalent to total knee replacement in terms of the knee-related quality of life as measured using the Oxford Knee Score after these two operations for patients with medial compartment osteoarthritis of the knee
Non-inferiority	Is the treatment non-inferior to the control?	To assess whether partial knee replacement is non-inferior to total knee replacement in terms of the knee-related quality of life as measured using the Oxford Knee Score after these two operations for patients with medial compartment osteoarthritis of the knee

Explanatory/pragmatic spectrum

Pragmatic Does the intervention treatment differ from the control in a typical clinical scenario?	 **PRECIS-2 domains** Eligibility criteria Recruitment Setting Organization Flexibility (delivery) Flexibility (adherence) Follow-up Primary outcome Primary analysis	**Explanatory** Does the treatment differ in an optimal scenario?
Impact on PICOTS P Patients thought to potentially benefit Intervention and Control are delivered according to centre and clinician practices Outcome of interest to patients and health professionals Time period is sufficient to observe completion of the current stage of the clinical pathway (e.g. unless treatment about further treatment is made) Setting is one which reflects typical clinical care		**Impact on PICOTS** P Patients thought to benefit the most Intervention and Control are delivered in a consistent approach between patients and across centres Outcome that confirms success (or not) of intervention treatment Time period is sufficient to observe early assessment of intervention and control effect Setting is one which is well suited to the intervention treatment

Related to this, the study tends to be more challenging to conduct. Perhaps most difficult are those where different types of treatment (e.g. a drug versus a surgical operation) are compared. For decisions related to the study design, the potential candidate options need to be considered in light of the research question and prior evidence. For example, if there are few safety data available on a new drug, we may be more inclined to opt for no control group in a phase 1 trial to maximize learning about the safety. Whereas, if the drug comes from a class of drugs for which the safety profile is well established, we may desire a control to allow a preliminary comparative assessment even at phase 1.

Outcome selection

The outcomes are the measures by which we quantify the effect of treatments. The data collected for them is then used in the statistical analysis to determine according to our study objectives what conclusions the data support. Outcomes come in a remarkably variety of shapes and forms, with lots of minor variations. Broadly, outcomes can be categorized as one of five types: critical events (e.g. death), clinical condition-specific status/biomarkers (e.g. recurrence of disease, or systolic blood pressure), health-related quality of life (whether overall, or with a restricted or condition-specific focus), patient satisfaction, knowledge or behaviour (e.g. would you recommend the treatment to others?), or healthcare usage (e.g. admission to hospital or further treatment). Outcome data may come from a variety of sources and types of assessment (e.g. the clinician's assessment of an MRI scan, patient questionnaires, and physical examinations). We will consider more about how we might collect the relevant data and the related challenges in Chapter 7.

Ultimately, we would like to select all the relevant types of outcomes which are of interest to any of the key stakeholders (patients, health professionals, regulatory, etc.). However, a particular clinical trial, especially earlier phase trials, may well only focus on a subset of the possibilities. The implicit expectation is that further studies will provide further evidence, and cover a greater range of outcomes. Safety of a drug treatment in particular, remains an area of interest even after the drug has become widely used. Some rare adverse events may only become apparent at a later point, and it may become clear that there are specific groups for whom this treatment is not appropriate. A key decision implicit in the formulation of the research question of a clinical trial is to clarify the type of outcome which will be the main focus in the evaluation. In particular, for the primary objective it should be clarified how this will be assessed and therefore what the main finding and interpretation of the study will be based upon. Typically, the associated outcome, the primary outcome, is the only one for which the study's sample size is directly tailored.

The lack of common outcomes across studies has been noted for years as a stumbling block to comparisons and syntheses of evidence across clinical trials. A review of 10,000 trials of schizophrenia treatments remarkably identified over 2000 different outcomes which was greater than the number of different treatments evaluated (10). The COMET (Core Outcome Measures in Effectiveness Trials) initiative provides a framework for ensuring common outcome types are collected for late phase trials. In a similar way, regulators and academic–industry collaborations such as OMERACT (Outcome Measures in Rheumatology) have gone some way to ensuring consistency of outcomes in future clinical trials. Nevertheless, more improvement is needed (11). A well-designed trial has a clear and coherent spine running from the study objectives through to the PICOTS elements. Therefore, clearly the primary outcome should be in keeping with the research question and the primary objective of the study. If the primary objective is to find the appropriate dose, then we would expect something like MTD to be the primary outcome. Similarly, if safety is also part of the primary objective we would in effect perhaps expect a type of safety outcome, measuring toxicity in some form, to be one of the key study outcomes, if not the primary outcome. Measuring the primary and any other key outcomes in a way that maintains comparability to any relevant existing studies should be the goal with a new measure or approach only preferred with appropriate justification.

Building the team

Clinical trials are perhaps the ultimate team science project. They require an increasing number of different competencies to be delivered. From the earliest days, the team or cooperative nature of delivering clinical trials was well recognized (12). It is not uncommon for large randomized phase 3 trials to involve more than 100 individuals at many different locations. Developing a clinical trial requires the formation of a core team who will generate a proposal to the level at which funding and appropriate regulatory approvals (e.g. healthcare system, ethical, and governmental authorities such as the MHRA and FDA) can be sought. The basic competencies required for developing a clinical trial are clinical or health professional, statistical, and study conduct. However, many studies will require clinicians with different specialisms; early phase drug trials will require pharmacology expertise and later phase trials may well require other academic disciplines such as health economics, qualitative research, and psychology among others. These expertise needs are increasingly filled not by a single individual but by two or more individuals to provide the oversight, range of expertise required, and sufficient capacity to deliver. The delivery aspect of trials will often require another layer of individuals to complement and supplement the team including recruitment specialists (often nurses), study coordination, data management, IT system, and administrative support and expertise. Accordingly, working with an established and experienced clinical trial group (e.g. typically called a clinical trials unit (CTU) in the UK, clinical research organization, or coordinating centre in the US) is often vital. Large pharmaceutical companies will have substantial in-house expertise in all aspects of clinical trials. Working with such a group shares a lot of the effort involved in developing an implementable and useful clinical trial. It also spares the lead investigators a lot of unnecessary pain in the early stages of development.

Developing a funding proposal

Clinical trials are time-consuming, complex, and demanding projects. As such, most will require an external funding source, sometimes involving a very substantial amount of money, to be conducted. Some small single-centre late phase clinical trials for non-drug treatments are still conducted with very limited funding. However, implicitly there is a lot of support being provided institutionally by the organizations the investigators work for and where the clinical trial will be conducted (e.g. universities and healthcare providers). Typically, a proposal will need to be made to secure funding for academic and clinically led proposals. A funding request may be made internally, such as within company structures in the pharmaceutical industry. Some form of co-funding is becoming more common with industry and public or charity funding. Different funding sources have different systems and peculiarities even among various funding streams from the same funder (e.g. such as the NIHR in the UK, the NIH in the US, and EU funding streams). The form of applications to these streams vary greatly. Nevertheless, the essence of a good proposal is consistent.

Four general points can be noted. First, a good funding proposal is one which falls within the remit of the funding call. This seems like an obvious point but as research starts with a question it is not always obvious who, or if anyone, will fund a study and it is certainly not a given it is appropriate for a particular funder, nor funding stream. Most funding streams from prospective funders will be tailored to different stages of research (e.g. early versus late clinical research), and sometimes to particular research areas (e.g. trauma) or even specific diseases (e.g. breast cancer). Second, a team with a track record has a particular advantage and in terms of delivery, linking with a group who have delivered clinical trials in the past, and ideally of a similar nature, is critical. Third, a good proposal is one where the research question and study design sit together coherently. Fourth, the proposal needs to be clearly written so that why the clinical trial is needed, what it will assess, how it will be conducted, and what it will achieve are clear, and it tells a compelling story.

Summary

Clarifying the research question of interest is the first step in designing a clinical trial. Both the PICOTS framework and the FINER criteria are helpful ways to clarify what is of most interest and how to assess the proposed research question in view of what is already known. The outline of research design and the research question intended to be addressed should be symbiotically related. Substantial adjustments in the design for whatever justifiable reason (e.g. changing the way the primary outcome will be measured) need to be considered in light of the research question posed. It is not uncommon to realize that once the design is considered in more depth, the research question will need tweaking as either it was ill posed, or modifying it would lead to a more coherent and addressable research question. Secondary and ancillary research questions can also be addressed through additional objectives though they must not be allowed to compromise the overall design. In some respects it could be said that one has never finished designing a study until it is completed. Nevertheless, the design which we start with is invariably the one we have to account for when the trial is over.

References

1. Evans SR. Fundamentals of clinical trial design. Journal of Experimental Stroke & Translational Medicine. 2010;3(1):19–27.
2. Borg Debono V, Zhang S, Ye C, Paul J, Arya A, Hurlburt L, et al. A look at the potential association between PICOT framing of a research question and the quality of reporting of analgesia RCTs. BMC Anesthesiology. 2013;13(1):44.
3. Rios LP, Ye C, Thabane L. Association between framing of the research question using the PICOT format and reporting quality of randomized controlled trials. BMC Medical Research Methodology. 2010;10:11.
4. Thabane L, Thomas T, Ye C, Paul J. Posing the research question: not so simple. Canadian Journal of Anaesthesia. 2009;56(1):71–9.

5. Schenk DB, Koller M, Ness DK, Griffith SG, Grundman M, Zago W, et al. First-in-human assessment of PRX002, an anti-α-synuclein monoclonal antibody, in healthy volunteers. Movement Disorders. 2017;32(2):211–18.

6. Beard DJ, Davies LJ, Cook JA, MacLennan G, Price A, Kent S, et al. Total versus partial knee replacement in patients with medial compartment knee osteoarthritis: the TOPKAT RCT. Health Technology Assessment. 2020;24(20):1–98.

7. Dawson J, Fitzpatrick R, Murray D, Carr A. Questionnaire on the perceptions of patients about total knee replacement. Journal of Bone and Joint Surgery British Volume. 1998;80(1):63–9.

8. Hulley SB, Cummings SR, Browner WS, Grady DG, Newman TB. Designing Clinical Research. Philadelphia, PA: Wolters Kluwer; 2013.

9. Loudon K, Treweek S, Sullivan F, Donnan P, Thorpe KE, Zwarenstein M. The PRECIS-2 tool: designing trials that are fit for purpose. BMJ. 2015;350:h2147.

10. Miyar J, Adams CE. Content and quality of 10 000 controlled trials in schizophrenia over 60 years. Schizophrenia Bulletin. 2012;39(1):226–9.

11. OMERACT. OMERACT. 2021. Available from: https://omeract.org/

12. Hill AB. The clinical trial. New England Journal of Medicine. 1952;247:113–19.

3
Randomized controlled trials

> To dismiss randomization with the remark, 'I don't need it', is amusing,
> perhaps, but in my serious judgment reflects an ignorance of scientific
> method in its general form. The simple answer to the question 'Who
> needs it' is 'My clients needs it'.
>
> **Oscar Kempthorne, 1977 (1)**

What is a randomized controlled trial?

There is only one unique feature of a randomized controlled trial (RCT): the
random allocation of the aspect under evaluation (typically the treatment received by a participant). Where treatments or other medical care interventions are randomly allocated, an RCT is also a clinical trial. Sometimes RCT
is accordingly spelt out as 'randomized clinical trial' in this setting to differ-
entiate such studies from RCTs in other contexts. However, the terminology
of 'randomized controlled trial' is the more common usage. Randomization
of treatments is the foundation upon which the RCT is built and by which related good scientific practices can be employed. It facilitates a fair, unbiased,
as statisticians or epidemiologists might call it, comparison of treatments. The
RCT is so much seen as the ideal or 'proper' clinical trial that the terms clinical
trial and RCT trial have been used interchangeably by even leading clinical
trialists (2). However, a number of the attractive design features of an RCT can
also be employed in other types of clinical trials (e.g. having a control group).
Correspondingly, randomization of treatments per se is far from sufficient on
its own.

The deceptively simple, yet often challenging to implement, difference of
randomly allocating the treatments leads to a number of profound implications and advantageous study attributes. These are summarized in Table 3.1.
First of all, randomization necessitates a prospective study. While clinical
trials under the definition in Chapter 1 must also be prospective in the sense
that they are 'planned' studies, it is important to note that many other types
of research studies are not. As a consequence, these studies are often not as

Table 3.1 Benefits arising from randomization in a randomized controlled trial

Benefit	Summary
Prospective	The study can be designed to collect all data required for the analysis and associated reporting
Consistent	Randomization is a study event for which the timing is known and the timing of randomization is planned. Clinical events can readily be identified as falling before or after randomization, and timed accordingly. Follow-up can be timed from randomization. Observational studies may not have all the relevant information to ensure consistency of timing among included individuals
Controlled	Randomization requires two or more options. Therefore, there will always be at least one reference (control) group to which a treatment group can be compared
Contemporary	As the allocation is random, the treatment groups are involved in the study in the same time period thus protecting against bias due to temporal trends (e.g. changes in clinical practice)
Comparable	The groups are anticipated to be similar due to random allocation and any imbalance is by chance
Analytic	Randomization justifies basic statistical analyses to compare the outcome between groups. It also provides a reference point from which the statistical properties of more complex analysis methods can be readily assessed

reliable or informative. Second, the point of randomization defines formal entry into the study; this might seem a minor point but it means that all participants have a common reference point from which *everything* that occurs to them can be gauged against, and follow-up can be timed consistently and impartially. Third, RCTs have a control group, hence the word 'controlled' in the name is unnecessary and 'randomized trial' is sometimes used instead. As we have seen in Chapter 1, some clinical trials, particularly early phase ones, may not have a control group. In contrast, an RCT always has a control providing a relevant reference group for comparison. Fourth, this randomized control is contemporary, that is, the period of time is the same as for the treatment group. Other studies may use patient data from what is called a historical control, that is, data from an earlier time period using data from the same or different sites. Therefore, any change in outcome over time (secular trend) may affect the measurement of the treatment effect inducing bias in such a comparison. Random allocation of treatment to patients over time protects the comparison from this. Fifth, the intervention and control groups will be comparable, or similar, prior to receipt of the treatment and at study entry. We will consider this point in more detail later in the chapter. Sixth, following on from the previous points, we therefore have a justification for a statistical analysis comparing intervention and control treatments given randomization has been carried out. We can quantify how unusual our observed findings are given we can reasonably expect the groups were the same initially. There is of course nothing stopping us from analysing data from any source in a similar way. Nevertheless, an RCT provide a 'safe space' to conduct statistical analyses with assurance. We will consider this point further in Chapter 9. Before proceeding, we will presume here that we are interested in allocating a series of individuals to receipt of a single treatment though that is not necessarily the case. We will consider some common variations in what is randomized in Chapter 4. Some of these (especially a cluster trial design) modify the way in which the benefits in Table 3.1 apply. This chapter will consider what makes the RCT a particularly valuable research design, before considering potential biases in how RCTs and other clinical trials are conducted. We will then look at what randomization achieves and how to randomize, before considering if RCTs are so great, why all clinical trials are not RCTs.

Why randomized controlled trials are the preferred research design for evaluating treatments

To understand the great interpretive power of random allocation it is helpful to consider the challenges of measuring the effect of a treatment. Intuitively, if we want to assess the effect of treatment, we could measure the outcome of interest after a patient has been treated. However, interpreting what to make of that single observation is more difficult than it might at first appear.

Suppose we gave a new chemotherapy treatment to a woman with stage 1 breast cancer and then assessed later whether the cancer had progressed or not. First, if it did not progress we might therefore be inclined to think that the new treatment did indeed work. However, what we do not know is what would have happened to her if she had not received this treatment. Might she have avoided progression by this point anyway? Furthermore, we also do not know if this outcome was certain to happen or just did in this case. Lastly, we might wonder if we were to give the treatment to other people whether it would it lead to the same finding. We know that different people can have different responses though we do not fully understand why. As we cannot assess the outcome more than once per person, we might therefore decide to measure the outcome for a group of people. Suppose we did this and out of 100 people the cancer in 30 (30%) did not progress. Should we conclude the new treatment works or not? The figure of 30% might well be viewed as disappointing on the face of it, but if without the new treatment the cancer did not progress in only 10% then we might well view this as a major success.

Accordingly, we would naturally therefore like to have another group of individuals to whom we do not give the new treatment to see if they differ. We will be able to compare them to the first group to see if the new treatment does indeed work better. We *can* attribute the difference between the new chemotherapy and control groups as being due to the treatment they have received *if one crucial condition holds*—that is, the two groups of people are the same except for the sole difference of which treatment they received. This is where randomization comes in as it gives us confidence that we have similar groups at the outset, and therefore reason to attribute the observed result (whether a positive, negative, or non-existent effect) to the treatment received.

It might be said that we could just treat some patients with the new chemotherapy treatment and then compare them against previous patients with the same condition. However, even if we assume that there have been no changes in clinical care, and that we have measured the outcome in the same way, we are still faced by a large assumption to make: namely that the two groups are the same in *all* regards. We could seek to get two groups which match for clinically important factors we know about. For example, we could measure things such as age, sex, disease status, and so on. Presuming that we can do this perfectly (which is for some characteristics much harder than it might at first seem), we still face the problem of potential differences in things we cannot measure, or know to be important but have no way to reliably and comprehensively quantify. These include quite subjective things such as the outlook of the patients, their lifestyle, and their diet, which are incredibly hard to measure in a reliable, comprehensive, and non-reductionist way. Perhaps most importantly, it also includes the major influence of genetics. We know that genetics influence the susceptibility to and progression of disease. It also affects the ability to recover yet we are incredibly far from being able to quantify and understand this for many individual diseases. Both the complexity of genetic data and the interwoven nature of genetics, lifestyle, and disease make it virtually impossible to ever fully untangle the causes of health outcomes. Fortunately we do not need to.

With random allocation of treatments to individuals we have the reassurance that the differences between the treatment groups are but random occurrences except for what occurs during the trial. As such, we can quantify how unusual the pattern of observed outcome data by treatment group is by using a statistical analysis. By randomizing we know that differences between the groups of both factors that we know matter to health outcome (e.g. age), and those we do not (such as specific genetic traits yet to be identified), differ at baseline (the beginning of the study), by random allocation alone.

Through the above example, simple and intuitive steps have led us, due to basic scientific principles, to conducting an RCT. An RCT can therefore reasonably be seen as the optimal scientific study to carry out when evaluating treatments. Many examples of the use of RCTs to evaluate treatments and the positive impact upon healthcare exist across medicine (2–6). However, we must note in passing that the RCT will need to be carried out in an appropriate manner for it to live up to this high reputation. We will consider this in more detail in this and later chapters.

The difficulties of interpreting the effect of a treatment

At the outset it is key to note that comparing the outcome in the two treatment groups in a controlled clinical trial helps us to determine the difference in outcome *between* the two treatments, not necessarily the effect that can be truly attributed to either treatment. Rarely, if ever, can we be confident that the effect we observed in a group receiving the same treatment can be fully attributed to the treatment concerned. There are four main, subtle but important, reasons for this. First, the natural course for the individual, driven by their personal characteristics, will make a substantial contribution (perhaps even the vast majority of the effect) towards their final outcome. This will be due to various factors including the influence of underlying genetics, and other patient characteristics such as age, biological sex, comorbidities, diet, and the lifestyle of individuals, as well as their disease status.

Second, medical care is often predicated upon an imperfect assessment of health. As such it is the more outlying observations, or extreme results (e.g. on a blood test), that tend to lead to treatment. Similarly, it is the point at which an individual feels worst that they seek care, and conversely, it is less common to do so if they are already well on the path to recovery. Therefore, there is reason to expect some return towards a more typical and healthy state irrespective of treatment received. This phenomenon has been called *regression to the mean* (7). It can occur in many different contexts and is one of the reasons why a control group, and a randomized controlled one in particular, is highly advantageous. The more extreme the measurement observed, the more regression towards the mean we may anticipate. For example, where eligibility to a clinical trial is explicitly linked to a measurement known to be imperfect, and to vary over time to a degree unrelated to the true underlying status (e.g. measurement error in taking the blood pressure for a trial of a drug for hypertension), regression to the mean will clearly occur.

Third, there is reason to believe that by carrying out a study and observing, we may well influence the outcome observed in unintended ways. Merely by the act of conducting the study and observing participants we may influence behaviour, and, therefore, the outcome. This has been referred to as the *Hawthorne effect* (8, 9). The name comes from a series of research studies of worker productivity conducted in the 1920s and 1930s in the Hawthorne Works factory in Illinois, US (9). Benefits in productivity and other outcomes initially attributed to changes in the workplace environment (such as changes to the lighting, supervision, and working day) were observed. However, these were latter argued to be due to the influence of conducting a study on the subjects and the workplace environment, and not, at least solely, to the interventions. Therefore, a Hawthorne effect might be defined as the effect of the experiment taking place upon the research participants and to their environment through knowledge of the study taking place or otherwise, which cannot be fairly attributed to the intervention of interest. Similarly, a 'clinical trial' effect has been suggested and observed whereby patients in the clinical trial appear to do somewhat better than corresponding patients outside the trial (10). This might reflect to a degree unplanned health benefits due to participation in a clinical trial.

Fourth, the act of intervening, and specifically giving a treatment, may carry with it a *placebo effect*. There may be some expectation by the individual receiving the treatment, which can influence the observed outcome which is not truly caused by the treatment itself, merely perceptions related to its receipt. This might influence their outcome in various ways. For example, it may make them more optimistic and therefore alter their behaviour in some way conducive to a better outcome (or merely to perceiving their outcome as such). The more orchestrated the treatment, perhaps the greater the placebo effect. In this way surgery might be seen to have the greatest placebo effect, as the process of receiving surgery is often following failed, initial, non-invasive treatments (e.g. pain management, rest, and physiotherapy), implying it is the 'stronger treatment'. Additionally, there is a whole process of preoperative and postoperative care associated with an operation (11). In an RCT comparing surgical versus medical management of gastro-oesophageal reflux disease, the knowledge of which treatment was to be received appeared to influence the perception of the participants' assessment of their own outcome, with those allocated to receive surgery perceiving themselves as less well than those allocated to medical management (12).

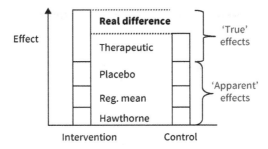

Figure 3.1 Anatomy of a treatment effect.
Note: Reg. mean, regression to the mean.

Therefore, there are a number of factors which make measurement of the attributable effect of treatments very difficult. However, with the use of randomization of treatment and associated procedures in the context of a well-conducted clinical trial, we can potentially address *all* of these factors. This allows isolation of an effect attributable to the choice of treatment. The benefits of the comparable control that randomization (and adequate associated strategies such as blinding) produces are shown visually in Figure 3.1. The measured effects of both the intervention and the control can be broken down into a number of contributing factors including the true effects of the treatments and 'apparent' (e.g. placebo, regression to the mean, and Hawthorne) effects.

An unbiased experiment

Scientifically we can state that we wish to compare the treatment groups in a way that ensures the assessment is fair and reliable. As we have considered above, creating similar groups is far from straightforward. With randomization of treatments we can prevent intentional and unintentional bias in the creation of the groups. We are likely to create similar groups, and at worst we have imbalance due to chance which we can reasonably adjust for statistically (13). However, randomization on its own is far from sufficient to ensure a fair experiment. What subsequently occurs can undermine the similarity of the groups in terms of the patient characteristics. Abel and Koch make this point, using a contrived example of the ultimate form of biased outcome assessment where they always give one treatment a better score than the other irrespective of any patient's response (14). While we would hope that this scenario is far from realistic, it does make the point that *randomization can be completely undermined by what occurs following allocation.* Implicitly, our consideration of the treatment effect above and the value attributed to randomization of treatment allocation presumes that this is not the case. However, for that to be true we need to design and conduct the RCT in an appropriate manner. Having determined how to randomize participants, and with the expectation of similar groups upon entry to the clinical trial, we now consider the delivery of the treatments and the follow-up (including data collection and outcome assessment). All aspects of the study need to be carefully planned to avoid introducing bias to one treatment over the other.

Many forms of bias can be identified. Sackett identified seven areas where some form of bias might be introduced into a research study from conception through to reporting (15). Figure 3.2 shows the flow of participants in a study and the key stages during the study at which common bias may be introduced into the comparison. The main ones in the context of conducting a clinical trial are often described as selection bias, performance bias, attrition bias, and detection bias (16). Further bias can be introduced at the reporting stage (see Chapter 10 for consideration of reporting). A well-designed RCT is one which seeks to minimize the threat, as far as possible, of these biases undermining the finding(s) of the study. The key aim is that what occurs subsequent to randomization is *identical except for that which we wish to compare* (i.e. the treatments).

We consider here in turn the four common forms of bias in designing and conducting an RCT using the Cochrane's risk of bias taxonomy (16). A more

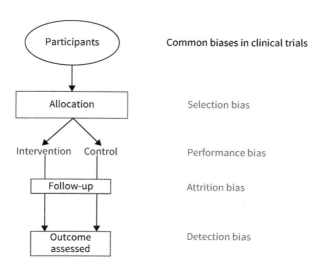

Figure 3.2 Patient flow and common biases in clinical trials.

elaborate approach to assessing bias could be adopted (indeed the version 2.0 of the Cochrane risk of bias tool has five domains and a slightly different formulation) (17). Here we use the simpler four bias structure to consider the potential influence of bias in the design and running of a RCT. First, we wish to avoid *selection bias*, that is, where groups are formed in a way which is favourable to one treatment over the other. The impact may be that any observed difference might be attributed to who is in the groups as opposed to the treatments. The use of randomization to allocate treatments to participants addresses this. Furthermore, the use of appropriate means to achieve allocation concealment, that is, concealing what future participants will be allocated to, preserves the benefit of random allocation of treatment, reducing or removing predictability.

Second, there may be *performance bias*, that is, bias in the way in which the treatments are to be implemented or some other aspects of care aside from the intrinsic difference which is the focus of the comparison. For example, if we were to have additional patient care, in terms of adjuvant care which could be given alongside both treatments but is only given to one group in practice, this could bias the comparison of the treatments. For example, in an RCT comparing two surgical procedures, the use of oral antibiotics to control potential for infections might be more common for one procedure than the other. This additional care may contribute to the observed difference between two treatments in terms of observed number of infections and associated outcomes. Therefore, how the treatments to be evaluated are delivered needs careful consideration. It is also worth noting that the setting is a related consideration and ultimately the design in this regard needs to match the research question. If those who receive the intervention treatment receive care in a different institution, such as a specialist hospital, whereas those who receive the control are looked after in their local hospital, this will have a substantial influence on a range of factors which can ultimately influence a range of outcomes. Perhaps a more likely issue in a clinical trial is not understanding the implications of providing both treatments in the local hospital or in the specialist centre. The setting will influence the staffing levels, equipment available, along with a range of local policies (e.g. use of adjuvant care, and discharge). These aspects need careful consideration.

The next main bias we wish to avoid or minimize is what is called *attrition bias*, that is, participants withdrawing from, or only partially completing, follow-up in a way which introduces bias to the comparison. For example, in clinical trials evaluating a drug treatment, it is not unusual for patients to cease treatment with the study drug when they experience a toxicity event or a severe adverse event. This is a natural response, and often entirely clinically appropriate. However, if their involvement in the study also ceases at that point, these individuals will not contribute to any later assessment of outcome which in turn could then be biased. Indeed, this may well perversely lead to bias in favour of this treatment with the greater pattern of drug-related toxicity (as those who drop out may well be those likely to have poorer outcomes). Therefore, the optimal, and desirable, position is that everyone who is randomized is followed up until the end of the study and all data are collected for them and included in the analysis. It is therefore not only the availability of data but its inclusion in the analysis which ultimately precludes attribution bias. We will consider this issue of who is analysed again in Chapter 9.

Lastly, we may have what has been called *detection bias*, that is, there is bias in the way which the outcomes are assessed which favours one group over the other. There are various ways in which this could occur in a study. These include the selection of a primary outcome which by definition favours one treatment over another. For example, some treatments can be repeated whereas others cannot (e.g. a simple comparison of further treatment will favour the one which cannot be repeated such as some surgical procedures). When the outcome is measured, it could favour one treatment over the other (e.g. it might be timed so as not capture the disadvantage of one treatment over another). Alternatively, how the outcome is assessed could also be a source of bias. For example, someone who is aware of the treatment received might unfairly assess subjective outcomes like symptoms less severely in one group than the other. Similarly, some adverse events are quite subjective in both their nature and severity and require careful clinical consideration of the specific details, and associated data such as imaging scans (e.g. identification of an occult hip fracture from an X-ray). As such, these assessments can be susceptible to conscious and unconscious bias.

A natural response to the possibility of detection bias might be to restrict the focus to more 'objective' outcomes for which the status can be more readily verified. However, often the outcomes which are most important to patients, and to an extent also health professionals, are by nature subjective. Symptoms such as pain, and someone's quality of life, are usually best assessed by the individual themselves. Therefore, some subjectivity in assessment is often inevitable and necessary. Accordingly, ensuring the assessor (whether the participant themselves or someone else) is not aware of which group the individual being assessed belongs to ('blind' to the treatment received) is often desirable. The ability to blind will depend greatly on the treatments being compared. Drug treatments are the easiest, that is not to say easy, to blind participants, care deliverers, and outcome assessors to, by using a placebo control. Physical placebos, such as surgery, are rarely used. In such a situation care needs to be taken to determine the intended mechanism of action (11). Blinded, or at least independent, outcome assessment though is usually possible, at least for some of the outcomes of interest (18). In addition to selection, performance, attribution and detection biases, we might also consider what is referred to *reporting bias*. Here the bias is due to selective, or misleading, presentation of the study findings. This type of bias can take various forms, and we will consider the issues related to reporting separately and more fully in Chapter 10. The above discussion is by no means intended to cover all possible 'bias' but to emphasise the more common areas of concern, and of the critical need to think through the design in light of this.

What does randomization achieve?

Having considered briefly the need to design and conduct the study overall in light of the research question and with the aim of minimizing bias, we now return to our consideration of randomization of treatment allocation, and what it achieves, in more detail (19). First, we have reason to expect our groups to be similar (thought it does not guarantee this if we are very unlucky with the allocations). In the negative sense, it prevents favouritism (whether intentional or accidental) towards one of the two groups when allocating. Thus, any imbalance which favours one group is by random chance and therefore, in principle, something which can be readily (if a relevant baseline measure is available) statistically adjusted for. Additionally, we are also not reliant on our understanding of the disease being treated to tell us what to control for when generating the groups. This strength has been clearly seen in the evaluation of potential treatments for COVID-19 where RCTs were able to assess whether a treatment worked even when our understanding of the disease was still at a fairly rudimentary level (20). The second thing it does, which is arguably purely the statistical representation of the first point, is that we have groups for which we can analyse statistically and quantify how unusual our observed data is. Our groups are thus statistically comparable as long as what subsequently occurs does not undermine this comparability. Third, due to randomization we can implement a number of desirable additional methodologies to address potential biases. We have discussed the main sources of bias earlier in this chapter; here we note the value of randomization is making the task of minimizing or avoiding them much easier. With randomization, as all participants have an equivalent starting point, we can implement identical care other than the aspect of care which we are evaluating. Furthermore, we can carry out the trial procedures, such as conducting follow-up and outcome assessment, in an identical and unbiased manner in the two groups. While not impossible in the absence of randomization, given limitations in data this is difficult to confidently assert as true or rectify as may be needed for observational studies using routine or retrospectively collected data. Lastly, as we have randomized, we can potentially conceal not only future allocations but also those which have already been received (i.e. undertake blinding). Who and for how long we might be able to or wish to do this for will vary between trials, but by randomizing it becomes a feasible option. Clearly, one does not wish to blind a surgeon to the operation they need to perform. However, it is not necessarily true that a participant in a clinical trial needs to immediately be aware of which treatment they have received, even sometimes surgery (5). We now consider the key issue of how to randomize and to do it in an appropriate way.

How to randomize

What needs to be achieved?

The full benefits of randomization are realized by the lack of certainty about which allocation a participant is going to receive. If we know what the next allocation is going to be then we could decide to recruit differently between the two groups. For example, we might select patients who are a little more likely to recover for the drug intervention group and a group who are somewhat less likely to recover for the control group. However, if it is a mystery to me, a 'random' occurrence of intervention or control, then I am no longer able to do this. To therefore be random, it needs to be both a fair allocation (generated using a method that is not prejudiced to one group over the other), and one which is unknown to those who are recruiting to the study. Therefore, we have three main tasks when carrying out randomization: (i) choosing an appropriate randomization method, (ii) generating the random sequence according to the chosen method, and (iii) delivering the random allocation in a way that preserves the benefits of the random sequence. We will consider these tasks in turn.

The main randomization options

There are three main types of randomization methods for an RCT: (i) simple randomization (i.e. without any constraint on the allocation of treatment other than the allocation ratio); (ii) restricted randomization, where the allocation is constrained either to achieve balance in group sizes, or balance in key characteristics of interest; and (iii) outcome-adaptive randomization, where randomization takes into account the known outcome and allocation received by previous participants. Some of the more common randomization methods belonging to each of the three main types are summarized in Table 3.2.

A key implicit decision when generating the allocation sequence is deciding upon the allocation ratio. In terms of both simplicity and from a statistical perspective (provided we anticipate similar variability in the outcome of interest in the two treatment groups), a fixed 1:1 allocation, that is, each treatment group has the same (50%) chance, is usually optimal. The sample size formulas we will see in Chapter 5 will assume this, and a 1:1 (equal chance) is overwhelmingly the most common practice in RCT with the standard design. However, it should be noted that we do not have to do so, and there are valid reasons why we might deviate from this, both practical (e.g. favouring one group might be thought to benefit recruitment), financial (e.g. if there is a substantial cost difference between the treatments the ratio could allow patients to be allocated more frequently to the cheaper treatment), and statistical (e.g. having a larger control group to increase statistical efficiency when more than one active treatment groups are used) (21). For example, in the phase 1 trial we considered in Chapter 1, most of the allocations were generated using a 5:1 ratio in favour of PRX002 drug over placebo (22). This meant more of the participants received the intervention drug, facilitating the varying of the dose level and the planned statistical analysis to explore the PK and PD of PRX002. Furthermore, we could proceed further and allow the ratio to vary from participant to participant depending upon outcome data on preceding participants (outcome-adaptive randomization). While such an approach is intuitively attractive, there are a number of limitations which have led to limited use of outcome-adaptive randomization. In short, the study may need to be substantially larger, and this approach may perversely lead to more individuals in the trial getting the inferior treatment. Extensive considerations of this issue can be found elsewhere along with examples (23,24).

It may surprise some readers how heated the debates regarding methods for randomization can be among statisticians. Some refer to certain approaches as 'proper' (e.g. simple) randomization against others such as minimization which can be fully deterministic (i.e. the next allocation is certain given that the preceding allocations and characteristics in the minimization algorithm are known). Alternatively, others have strongly advocated for minimization even as the 'platinum standard' (25). Some would argue for simple randomization over more complex methods for a range of reasons (26).

Table 3.2 Common randomization methods with examples

Name (type)	Description	Example text	Advantages	Disadvantages
Simple (unrestricted)	Participants are allocated with the same probability (typically 1 in 2) of being in each group. Each participant's allocation is completed separately (i.e. is not related to the allocation of any other participants) and is not related to any characteristics of that individual	'Patients were randomly assigned (1:1) by simple randomisation to the SMS intervention or to standard care (control group). A project statistician generated the randomisation numbers with a random number generating program. Written allocation of assignment was sealed in individual opaque envelopes marked with study identification numbers, which were distributed to all three study clinics' (30)	• Straightforward to carry out • Does not necessarily require the allocations to be generated in advance (though this is often done) • Easier to maintain allocation concealment as long as those recruiting do not generate the allocation, or have access to the allocation sequence	• Likely but does not guarantee control on the size of the groups • Key characteristics could be substantially imbalanced between groups
Random permuted block (restricted)	Participants' allocations are generated in blocks with a random order (e.g. sets of four allocations) to ensure the desired balance of allocations	'... eligible patients were enrolled through a web-based system established for this trial and randomized by a computer-generalized permuted block sequence. The size of the blocks used for randomization was 4. The principal surgeons received a randomly generated assignment (1:1) allocating the patients to one of the 'closure' groups' (31)	• Fairly simple to carry out • Ensures similar group sizes (equal if all blocks are completed)	• Allocations need to be generated in advance (at least the block but typically the full set) • If the previous allocations, the current block size and the position in the block, and allocation ratio are known, the last allocation (sometimes others) in the block can be determined. To make it more difficult to predict future allocations, variable blocks sizes can be used

| Stratification with random permuted blocks (restricted) | Participants are sorted into strata according to one or more characteristics (such as age, sex, and disease severity). Allocations within all possible combinations of characteristics subtypes are carried out separately | 'Randomization codes were produced by means of the PROC PLAN of the SAS system, with a 1:1 assignment ratio, stratifying by centre and using blocks multiple of 2 elements. The randomization schedule will be managed through the eCRF [electronic case report form] in a concealed manner' (32)

'Randomisation was done via an interactive voice and web response system using a permuted block scheme (block size of six) and was stratified by PD-L1 status, world region, and liver metastases' (33)

'Immediately after completing the baseline assessment, participants will be randomly allocated to either the walking and education programme (intervention) or no treatment (control) group. Randomisation using a 1:1 allocation ratio will be conducted using a schedule that has been pre-generated by an online programme, by an investigator not involved in participant recruitment or assessment. Randomisation will use randomly permuted blocks of 4, 6 and 8 and be stratified by history of >2 previous lifetime episodes of LBP (known to be a prognostic factor for recurrence), and recruitment from the community or clinician referral' (34) | • Constrains randomization to ensure one or more factors are well balanced
• Allocations within each factor level are independent of each other and therefore allocation concealment is not undermined | • Stratification factor level data need to be available at the time of randomizing
• Implementation is more complex. Requires an approach which will ensure balance according to the stratification factor levels. Typically conducted with random permuted blocks to ensure similar group sizes and therefore also has the same limitations (needs to be generated in advance, and potential for future allocations to be known)
• Only a limited number of characteristics and levels within them can realistically be controlled for. A separate list is required for every combination of stratification levels. For example stratifying for two factors each with 3 levels required 3x3=9 separate randomisation lists. |

(continued)

Table 3.2 Continued

Name (type)	Description	Example text	Advantages	Disadvantages
Minimization (restricted)	Participants are allocated in a way so as to reduce ('minimize') imbalance in one or more characteristics given previous allocations and the respective characteristics of those randomized so far. The basic approach (Taves) has two steps: (i) For the two treatment groups in turn, sum across the minimization factors the number of individuals in that group who have the same level for each factor as the individual to be allocated (ii) Allocate to the treatment group with the lower tally. If there is a tie then randomly allocate using simple randomization A common addition is to incorporate a 'random twist' whereby the allocation according to minimization as above is used most but not all of the time (e.g. 80% of the time) with participants receiving the treatment with the higher tally the remaining portion of the time	'Eligible patients were randomly assigned (1:1) to receive either first-line mFOLFOX6 plus bevacizumab followed by FOLFIRI plus bevacizumab after disease progression (control group), or first-line FOLFOXIRI plus bevacizumab followed by reintroduction of the same regimen after disease progression (experimental group). Randomisation was done using a centralised web-based system with a minimization algorithm to obtain balanced assignment in each treatment group according to the stratification factors: treatment centre, ECOG performance status (0 vs 1–2), primary tumour location (right-sided vs left-sided or rectum) and previous exposure to an adjuvant treatment (yes vs no). The random allocation sequence was masked and was generated at the Clinical Trials Coordinating Center, Istituto Toscano Tumori (Florence, Italy)' (35)	• Constrains randomization to ensure one or more factors are well balanced • Ability to handle a larger number of factors simultaneously even in smaller studies	• The next allocation is knowable if the previous allocations and characteristics are known along with the specific minimization algorithm used. To make this more difficult, a 'random twist' is sometime used where allocation follows simple randomization instead of minimization for a small proportion of the time. Additionally, simple randomization may be used initially to 'seed' the allocation list prior to starting to use minimization • Use of minimization for trials with greater than two arms or to implement unequal allocation ratios requires particular care • Minimization system needs careful checking to avoid errors

Bayesian outcome adaptive randomization (outcome-adaptive randomization)

Participants are allocated taking into account the outcome of preceding participants. The probability of being allocated to the treatment groups is based upon the probability of the corresponding treatment having the better outcome. A common formula (23) used to calculate the probability of randomizing to treatment group I (intervention group) given current data (D) is:

$$\frac{\Pr(I > C \mid D)^W}{\Pr(I > C \mid D)^W + (1 - \Pr(I > C \mid D))^W}$$

where $\Pr(I > C \mid D)$ refers to the probability that the outcome in the intervention group (I) is greater than the outcome in control group (C) given the data accumulated at the point of randomization. W is a constant which can be varied to alter the characteristics of allocation. If W = 0 it is sometimes referred to a 'play the winner' randomization. W = 0.5 is also commonly used (36). The calculation of the probabilities is done under a Bayesian framework, and varies according to the analysis of the outcome

'The primary study objective was to assess and compare the efficacy of clofarabine alone versus clofarabine plus low-dose cytarabine. Patients were adaptively randomized without stratification factors. Assignment probabilities were based on the observed results in the preceding patients, according to the method of Berry (Bayesian randomization). For the first 20 patients, the randomization was balanced with a 50% probability of being randomized to either arm. As data accrued concerning efficacy, the assignment probabilities shifted in favor of the arm with a higher CR rate. Information on each patient's response was entered using a web-based data entry screen that was provided by the Department of Biostatistics at the MDACC' (37)

- Could be viewed as more ethical as a participant's chance of receiving the best treatment follows the accumulating evidence
- Can be readily extended to incorporate a 'stopping rule' to determine if a treatment is not suitable for randomization

- Each allocation requires data from previous individuals to be collected and analysed. This requires a quick and robust system of data collection and statistical analysis. The outcome also needs to be one which can be assessed in a short time frame
- Allocation probabilities are volatile in the early part of the trial where outcome data for only a few participants are available. Given this, simple randomization may be used initially to 'seed' the allocation list prior to using outcome-adaptive allocation
- The approach is susceptible to bias if participants' characteristics change over time
- It does not allocate in a statistically efficient way and may not provide sufficient data to quantify treatment effect

On the face of it, it can be argued that simple randomization is entirely sufficient if implemented using a safe approach (e.g. the randomization schedule is not produced either in advance or on demand by someone who is recruiting or treating patients, and it is kept separate from these individuals). Nevertheless, the concern of being particularly 'unlucky' for a specific trial (with an extreme imbalance in the numbers in each group and their key characteristics) tends to lead to some form of restricted randomization being used even though in terms of statistical precision the loss is very likely to be modest (26). For example, if we have a trial of 60 participants with a standard design, and using simple randomization and 1:1 allocation we have a 1 in 100 chance of imbalance in group sizes of 2:1. This results in a loss of only 6% statistical precision with a continuous primary outcome assuming equal variances and normally distributed data as is typically done in a standard analysis (e.g. t-test). More problematic for smaller trials is the potential inability to adjust the analysis reliably for baseline variables of interest and to carry out subgroup analyses where there is substantial imbalance in treatment group sizes. More important than strict numerical balance is imbalance in key prognostic factors at baseline which might casts some doubt upon the validity of findings. However, this can typically be addressed in the analysis though use of adjustment (e.g. use of a regression model in the analysis). Multiple analyses might be needed, possibly leading some to cast doubt upon the interpretation if the results of these analyses disagree.

Choosing an appropriate randomization method

There are a number of possible randomization method options and therefore their appropriateness needs to be considered in light of what is known about the condition, the treatments to be evaluated, the setting in which the study is going to be conducted, and the study design to be used. A few general principles can be outlined:

Use of a restricted randomization method should be related to its potential impact upon statistical efficiency and predictability, and not an esoteric view of what is truly 'random'. All computer-generated allocation methods, strictly speaking, are pseudo-random though some are much easier to make unpredictable to external parties (and to the person producing the allocations). Even simple randomization can lack allocation concealment if not implemented correctly. It is important to conceal as much as possible the specifics of the process by which the allocations are generated (and particularly the list of allocations if this is produced in advance). For example, in an RCT of two ways to conduct breast cancer screening, the algorithm used to generate the allocations according to simple randomization was concealed to all but one investigator in order to maintain allocation concealment (27). Such an individual should not be involved in recruitment or treatment of participants.

The smaller the number of individuals to be randomized, the greater the potential need for restricted randomization as appropriate adjustment in the statistical analysis will be more difficult (26). The possibility of a very statistically inefficient imbalance in the numbers in each group is much more likely for small studies. In a study of, say, 60 compared to a trial of 1000, an imbalance of 2:1 in the group sizes will have a much greater impact upon statistical precision and analysis options (e.g. groups of 20 and 40 versus 333 and 667).

Controlling a factor in the randomization should generally only be considered if it is known to be prognostically related to outcome. Inclusion of factors which are not prognostically related is unnecessary, and if only weakly related, imbalance, even if severe, is unlikely to matter. For example, controlling for baseline blood pressure levels makes sense in a trial of drug treatments for hypertension. A larger study will be expected to have a smaller magnitude of imbalances between baseline factors (including those which are prognostic). However, it is worth noting that a larger study per se is not protective against the adverse effect of covariate imbalance in terms of testing for a difference in the statistical analysis (13). The most noteworthy exception to the principle presented of controlling only for factors believed to be prognostically related is study centre, which is often controlled for in the randomization. The centre a participant belongs to can indicate a wide range of factors which together we might wish to control for various reasons (not only if we believe there to be a direct prognostic influence on the primary outcome).

The number of factors controlled for, if any, should be kept to a minimum. Each factor included in the randomization method (e.g. either by stratifying on it or incorporating in minimization) increases the complexity of the randomization process. This increases the likelihood of errors either in the generation of the allocations or in providing the correct information (25,28,29). Furthermore each factor controlled for in the randomization method (e.g. used to stratify for) should preferably be adjusted for in the statistical analysis to maintain appropriate statistical precision.

The allocation methods will need to be implemented in a suitable way to deliver the allocation as and when needed. Only factors for which the value will be readily available at the intended time of randomization can be accounted for. Treatments related to surgery are an interesting special case where randomization would ideally often occur immediately preceding or even during surgery. Nevertheless, for practical reasons, and due to the management of patient care, the preferred approach may not be possible. The point at which randomization is to take place will often impact what clinical information is routinely available. Additional data may need to be collected as part of the clinical trial, or some options may not be practical to implement even if the data could in theory be available. For example, the final surgical assessment of patient suitability and the extent of disease are often made during surgery as preoperative physical assessments and imaging have limitations. Prior to the operation a preliminary assessment which leads to the decision to operate and conduct a specific procedure is taken, but this is confirmed once the operation has begun. Therefore, randomization prior to the operation which is convenient for various practical reasons (including preparing the equipment, patient consent, etc.) would mean the final assessment of disease status cannot then be controlled for in the randomization method.

Generating the allocation sequence

In this section we will consider in turn some of the more commonly used allocation methods (simple, stratified with random permuted blocks, and minimization). For ease of presentation, we will consider only a two-arm RCT in which participants receive a randomly even (1:1) allocation to one of two treatments, the intervention (I) or the control (C).

Simple randomization: this could in theory be implemented for even (1:1) allocation by tossing a coin. However, the early 20th century RCTs predating the computer age often used a preprepared sequence of random numbers to generate the random sequence of treatment allocations. Figure 3.3 gives an example of how a table of random numbers varying from 0 to 9 can be used to divide the participants into two groups, which we would expect to be roughly evenly sized. The simple rule of using odd numbers for the intervention treatment (I) and even numbers for allocation to the control group (C) is used and applied to the participants. More commonly today, the sequence is generated from random numbers using a computer rather than by hand using random number tables (38). This could all be done in advance, that is, a sufficiently long list with a sequence of allocations is computer generated at the outset, or at the time of randomization the next allocation could be generated. How difficult the generation of the next allocation is and how far in advance, if at all, the sequence can be produced depend upon the randomization method used. For simple randomization and random permuted block allocation the list can be generated in advance as shown in Figure 3.3. Where the sequence is generated in advance, a check can be carried out on

Simple randomization using a list of
random numbers (0–9)

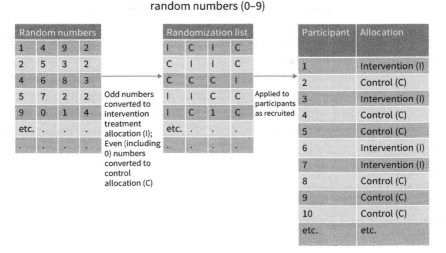

Random numbers					Randomization list					Participant	Allocation
1	4	9	2		I	C	I	C			
2	5	3	2		C	I	I	C		1	Intervention (I)
4	6	8	3		C	C	C	I		2	Control (C)
5	7	2	2		I	I	C	C		3	Intervention (I)
9	0	1	4		I	C	I	C		4	Control (C)
etc.	.	.	.		etc.	.	.	.		5	Control (C)
.	.	.	.		.	.	.	.		6	Intervention (I)
										7	Intervention (I)
										8	Control (C)
										9	Control (C)
										10	Control (C)
										etc.	etc.

Odd numbers converted to intervention treatment allocation (I); Even (including 0) numbers converted to control allocation (C)

Applied to participants as recruited

Figure 3.3 Simple randomization using a random number table.

the relative size of the allocation groups. We could choose to reject sequences with extreme imbalances under simple randomisation. However, excluding sequences generated in this way is akin to using a form of restricted randomization even if the list was originally generated without any restriction. The published literature suggests some form of selecting sequences is routinely done in practice where 'simple' randomisation has been used. It would be better to do such selecting in a formal way so that we can understand the implications. A similar but more formal approach would be to randomise the order of a fixed number of intervention and control treatments to be allocated to participants (e.g. for a trial of 100 participants, a sequence containing 50 interventions and 50 controls in a random order could be generated). As long as the target is reached the groups will be similarly sized. There is also a class of randomization methods which directly impose a minimal level of restriction to ensure the imbalance in group sizes at any point in the sequence is below a certain size; these are called maximally tolerated imbalance methods (39). However, these methods are more complex to implement, and we do not consider these any further here. The simplest approach to maintaining balance in the group sizes throughout the sequence is to use random permuted block allocation. Under this approach we just need to ensure we allocate in set of allocations (blocks) which have an even (for a 1:1 allocation) number of allocations to the two groups. A check of a sequence generated under block randomisation would then be solely for the purpose of ensuring the block randomisation was carried out appropriately. We will see how this works as we consider stratification, as this approach is usually used to implement stratified randomization.

Stratification (with random permuted blocks): the use of stratification is illustrated in Figure 3.4 where stratification on the basis of one factor, biological sex (male or female), is used. Using random permuted blocks this equates to having two separate randomization lists generated using random permuted blocks, one for men and one for women. The next unused allocation is taken according to the sex of the participant. In this example we show only 12 participants being randomly allocated which would be a very small clinical trial. Three points are worth noting. First, the number used from each list is dependent upon the sex split of the participants. Here there are four men and eight women, therefore we used the corresponding number of allocations from the prepared list for men and women (as shown in bold). Second, the final list also depends upon the order of the participants turning up. If the same 12 participants turned up but in a different order, the sequence would be shuffled accordingly; however, the same 12 allocations would be used. Third, as we have completed the blocks (in the figure each line represents a block) the final allocations are neatly balanced, that is, we have the same number of men and women in treatment groups A and B. However, this will often not be the case, and we can have a noticeable difference in the overall number of

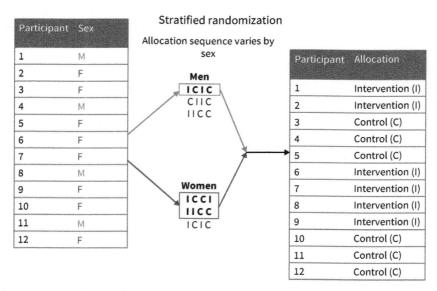

Figure 3.4 Stratified randomization example.
Note: this example uses a fixed block size of four. However, blocks can be of any size, and varying the block size is often used to further obscure future allocations (i.e. maintain allocation concealment).

individuals allocated to each treatment group. This depends upon how many individuals have been randomized, the stratification factors being used, the stratification characteristics of the randomized participants, and the size of the blocks within the strata combination. The greater the number of stratification factors and levels within, the higher this imbalance can be (though this will typically still be very modest compared to the overall size of the study).

Minimization: this method proceeds in a similar manner to stratification but instead of having a separate list for each combination of factor levels, like stratification does, the characteristics of the previously randomized participants are used to determine the allocation of the next participant, which would lead to the least (i.e. minimizing) imbalance with regard to these factors. There are various forms of minimization that have been proposed (and some similar, arguably statistically more desirable, but also more complex methods). However, the method by Taves appears to be the most commonly used one (25). We illustrate using the example above but instead of controlling only for biological sex we also control for age as well with two age groups (50 years and above or under 50 years old). Table 3.3 shows the calculations for participants 1–12 in a hypothetical trial. For at least the first allocation, and any subsequent ones where there is a tie, the randomization is made with simple randomization (indicated with '(random)' in the final allocation column). If we consider the third patient to be allocated, we can see that they are female and in the 50 years old or over age group. Of the previous allocations only one was a woman and only one was in the same age group (in this case the same patient, no. 2) who was allocated to group B. Therefore, the total for group A is 0 but the total for group B is 2. This means that the allocation according to minimization is group A. Of the 12 patients allocated happily we end up with six allocated to group A and six allocated to group B. By sex we have two men and four women in each group, and by age we have two in each group who are under 50 years old and four in each group who are 50 years or older.

Delivering the treatment allocations

We now consider how we can deliver the treatment allocations when running our RCT. There are three common ways in which the randomized allocation can be delivered: (i) use of an instantaneous allocation method by the recruiter (e.g. pre-prepared envelopes), (ii) allocation conducted at a separate location and communicated to the centre (e.g. at the trial office, see Chapter 8), and (iii) use of an individual or group within the centre where the trial is running to provide the allocation when needed (e.g. a member of pharmacy staff in

Table 3.3 Minimization example

Patient	Sex	Age (years)	Total with similar characteristics in intervention group = no. in sex group + no. in age group	Total with similar characteristics in control group = no. in sex group + no. in age group	Allocation which will minimize imbalance	Final allocation
1	M	37	0 + 0 = 0	0 + 0 = 0	Tie	Intervention (random)
2	F	72	0 + 0 = 0	0 + 0 = 0	Tie	Control (random)
3	F	51	0 + 0 = 0	1 + 1 = 2	Intervention	Intervention
4	M	60	1 + 1 = 2	0 + 1 = 1	Control	Control
5	F	78	1 + 1 = 2	1 + 2 = 3	Intervention	Intervention
6	F	47	2 + 1 = 3	1 + 0 = 1	Control	Control
7	F	66	2 + 2 = 4	2 + 2 = 4	Tie	Control (random)
8	M	61	1 + 2 = 3	1 + 3 = 4	Intervention	Intervention
9	F	55	2 + 3 = 5	3 + 3 = 6	Intervention	Intervention
10	F	69	3 + 4 = 7	3 + 3 = 6	Control	Control
11	M	45	2 + 1 = 3	1 + 1 = 2	Control	Control
12	F	37	3 + 1 = 4	4 + 2 = 6	Intervention	Intervention

Note: the allocation suggested by the minimization algorithm is given as well as the final allocation provided. The text '(random)' in the final allocation column indicates that the allocation was based upon a simple randomization to determine which group to allocate to. This was used where the minimization algorithm produced a 'Tie' (i.e. the tally for the two treatment groups were the same).

a hospital). With each of these approaches different methods can be used to produce and communicate the allocation to the relevant individual at the site.

Simple randomization (1:1) could be performed when needed, for example, by a coin-toss. This requires only the coin to be available to the person requiring the allocation and is very convenient and has been used. In the recent past a designated 'on-call' randomizer was used in some trials to provide an out-of-hours randomization service (so as to avoid such a problem). Fortunately, with advances in technology and the explosion of internet access and mobile phones, automated randomization systems with options of telephone or webpage access can make randomization readily available whenever needed (24 hours a day, 365 days a year). In choosing the mode of delivery there are a number of considerations. First, it must work with our chosen randomization method, for example, we cannot use a simple list of sealed envelopes as our method of delivery if we wish to use minimization as the next allocation is dependent upon the characteristics of the patients allocated so far. Second, methods which enable tracking of the allocations and therefore assessment of potential misuse are to be preferred. Use of a coin, drawing lots, and so on can be repeated without any record until the desired allocation is produced (or perhaps not even done in the first place). In contrast, computer automated systems can log when the randomization was conducted, or at least attempted. Relevant details can be collected at the time of randomization (e.g. stratification factor levels), and who requested the allocation can also be recorded. Third, we wish to use an approach which prevents knowledge of future allocations as this might facilitate the undermining of the allocation via selective recruitment to the study. The key point here is not so much which method is used but that the recruiter and those who treat patients do not have access to the allocations before they are assigned to a participant. Randomization and storage of allocations by an external party, whether a statistician at a trial office or through the use of an automated and secure randomization system, is highly desirable. Fourth, we want randomization to be possible *whenever* needed. Therefore, automated, computerized systems which are available 24 hours a day, 7 days a week without requiring a third party to be available are the optimal approach, particularly for studies running across multiple sites. If the low-tech option of a set of envelopes each with an allocation inside them is to be used, a couple of precautions are needed: (i) the envelopes need to be sealed and opaque so that the future allocations cannot be readily known and (ii) they should also be sequentially numbered so that any breaks in the order can be detected.

Why are all clinical trials not randomized controlled trials?

Given the discussion above, it might be taken for granted that all clinical trials should be RCTs. Indeed, as noted earlier, so strong was this view that some authors have used the terms clinical trial, controlled clinical trial, and RCT fairly interchangeably as a 'proper' clinical trial will have a control and the most appropriate control is a randomized one (2). Nevertheless, many clinical trials are *not* RCTs. Outside of the regulatory environment, there are many studies which are in essence a clinical trial, and purport to address a research question about the choice of treatments, but do not use an RCT design. Much can be said about this issue, but we restrict the focus here to a short summary of common reasons why randomization may not be used. First, randomization may be unnecessary as the objective can be achieved without it. For example, dose escalation or a very preliminary safety assessment can be made only on the treated participants. Randomization is needed for comparative assessment but that could come in later studies. Second, and for evaluations of non-drug treatments such as surgery, it can be viewed as 'too early' to assess with an RCT as the treatment may still be undergoing refinement, or expertise with it may be being gained (5). Third, an RCT might be viewed as 'unethical' in a particular scenario. Randomization is predicated upon sufficient uncertainty in the benefits and risks of the treatments to which participants are to be randomized. Where that is the case, it might even be argued randomization is more ethical as everyone will have a chance of receiving the optimal treatment. However, if this uncertainty is lacking, whether among potential participants, or health professionals, it cannot proceed even if desired. Some go so far as to question whether such 'equipoise' about the treatments can ever truly exist though strong counter arguments to this point have been made. The concept of clinical (or community) equipoise has been proposed to describe the corporate level, and to clarify how a health professional might participate even when they have a preference or belief in which treatment works best (40). Nevertheless, it certainly appears to be true that addressing specific research questions with an RCT, at times, may not be appropriate given what is already known. It is worth noting this judgement could change over time, both in favour of, and against, conducting an RCT. Fourth, randomization may not be feasible to address some research questions, even some related to the evaluation of specific treatments. Use of randomization leads to increased regulatory burden and requires greater resources to deliver. This cost (monetary or personnel capacity related) may be prohibitive. Alternatively, while we might in principle view the RCT as appropriate, there may not be sufficient acceptance in practice to conduct it. This could be because the burden of conducting the trial is felt to be too onerous (e.g. alongside clinical commitments or the demand upon patients is substantial). Then again, it might be the case that the allocation options in the randomization are not ones that a sufficient number of individuals will consent to in a reasonable time period. For example, the allocated treatments may differ greatly in a way which attracts and repels individuals (e.g. surgery versus oral drug treatment for a chronic condition such as severe osteoarthritis). Alternatively, it may not be possible to carry out a large enough RCT to evaluate some outcomes of interest (e.g. very rare safety events). Therefore for scientific, ethical and practical reasons, a RCT design may well not be the most appropriate design for some situations even when the overarching purpose is the evaluation of a treatment.

Summary

RCTs are the preferred design for a clinical trial which seeks to compare the outcome between treatments. Randomization naturally leads to a number of related features of good scientific practice which together facilitate a comparison which allows for quantification of the treatment effect. Like all studies, RCTs can be susceptible to bias and need to be designed and conducted carefully. Randomization can be carried out in a number of different ways. The choice of randomization method requires careful consideration of the setting and current knowledge about the condition of interest and how the random allocations will be generated and delivered in practice.

References

1. Kempthorne O. Why randomize? Journal of Statistical Planning and Inference. 1977;1(1):1–25.
2. Doll R. Clinical trials: retrospect and prospect. Statistics in Medicine. 1982;1(4):337–44.
3. Meldrum ML. A brief history of the randomized controlled trial. From oranges and lemons to the gold standard. Hematology/Oncology Clinics of North America. 2000;14(4):745–60.
4. Peto R. Reflections on the design and analysis of clinical trials and meta-analyses in the 1970s and 1980s. Journal of the Royal Society of Medicine. 2019;112(2):78–80.
5. Cook JA. The challenges faced in the design, conduct and analysis of surgical randomised controlled trials. Trials. 2009;10:9.
6. 2 Minute Medicine. The Classics in Medicine™: summaries of the landmark trials. 2022. Available from: https://www.2minutemedicine.com/the-classics-directory/
7. Morton V, Torgerson DJ. Effect of regression to the mean on decision making in health care. BMJ. 2003;326(7398):1083–4.
8. McCarney R, Warner J, Iliffe S, van Haselen R, Griffin M, Fisher P. The Hawthorne effect: a randomised, controlled trial. BMC Medical Research Methodology. 2007;7:30.
9. Olson R, Verley J, Santos L, Salas C. What we teach students about the Hawthorne studies: a review of content within a sample of introductory I-O and OB textbooks. The Industrial-Organizational Psychologist. 2004;41:23–39.
10. Braunholtz DA, Edwards SJ, Lilford RJ. Are randomized clinical trials good for us (in the short term)? Evidence for a 'trial effect'. Journal of Clinical Epidemiology. 2001;54(3):217–24.
11. Beard DJ, Campbell MK, Blazeby JM, Carr AJ, Weijer C, Cuthbertson BH, et al. Considerations and methods for placebo controls in surgical trials (ASPIRE guidelines). Lancet. 2020;395(10226):828–38.
12. Grant A, Wileman S, Ramsay C, Bojke L, Epstein D, Sculpher M, et al. The effectiveness and cost-effectiveness of minimal access surgery amongst people with gastro-oesophageal reflux disease—a UK collaborative study. The REFLUX trial. Health Technology Assessment. 2008;12(31):1–181.
13. Senn SJ. Covariate imbalance and random allocation in clinical trials. Statistics in Medicine. 1989;8(4):467–75.

14. Abel U, Koch A. The role of randomization in clinical studies: myths and beliefs. Journal of Clinical Epidemiology. 1999;52(6):487–97.

15. Sackett DL. Bias in analytic research. Journal of Chronic Diseases. 1979;32(1–2):51–63.

16. Mansournia MA, Higgins JP, Sterne JA, Hernán MA. Biases in randomized trials: a conversation between trialists and epidemiologists. Epidemiology. 2017;28(1):54–9.

17. Higgins JPT, Savović J, Page MJ, Sterne JAC on behalf of the RoB2 Development Group. Revised Cochrane risk-of-bias tool for randomized trials (RoB 2). 2019.

18. Boutron I, Guittet L, Estellat C, Moher D, Hróbjartsson A, Ravaud P. Reporting methods of blinding in randomized trials assessing nonpharmacological treatments. PLoS Medicine. 2007;4(2):e61.

19. Armitage P. The role of randomization in clinical trials. Statistics in Medicine. 1982;1(4):345–52.

20. RECOVERY Collaborative Group. Dexamethasone in hospitalized patients with Covid-19. New England Journal of Medicine. 2021;384(8):693–704.

21. Peckham E, Brabyn S, Cook L, Devlin T, Dumville J, Torgerson DJ. The use of unequal randomisation in clinical trials—an update. Contemporary Clinical Trials. 2015;45(Pt A):113–22.

22. Schenk DB, Koller M, Ness DK, Griffith SG, Grundman M, Zago W, et al. First-in-human assessment of PRX002, an anti-α-synuclein monoclonal antibody, in healthy volunteers. Movement Disorders. 2017;32(2):211–18.

23. Korn EL, Freidlin B. Outcome-adaptive randomization: is it useful? Journal of Clinical Oncology. 2011;29(6):771–6.

24. Grieve AP. Response-adaptive clinical trials: case studies in the medical literature. Pharmaceutical Statistics. 2017;16(1):64–86.

25. McPherson GC, Campbell MK, Elbourne DR. Investigating the relationship between predictability and imbalance in minimisation: a simulation study. Trials. 2013;14:86.

26. Hewitt CE, Torgerson DJ. Is restricted randomisation necessary? BMJ. 2006;332(7556):1506–8.

27. Hofvind S, Holen ÅS, Aase HS, Houssami N, Sebuødegård S, Moger TA, et al. Two-view digital breast tomosynthesis versus digital mammography in a population-based breast cancer screening programme (To-Be): a randomised, controlled trial. Lancet Oncology. 2019;20(6):795–805.

28. Yelland LN, Sullivan TR, Voysey M, Lee KJ, Cook JA, Forbes AB. Applying the intention-to-treat principle in practice: guidance on handling randomisation errors. Clinical Trials. 2015;12(4):418–23.

29. Strecher VJ, McClure JB, Alexander GL, Chakraborty B, Nair VN, Konkel JM, et al. Web-based smoking-cessation programs: results of a randomized trial. American Journal of Preventive Medicine. 2008;34(5):373–81.

30. Lester RT, Ritvo P, Mills EJ, Kariri A, Karanja S, Chung MH, et al. Effects of a mobile phone short message service on antiretroviral treatment adherence in Kenya (WelTel Kenya1): a randomised trial. Lancet. 2010;376(9755):1838–45.

31. Imamura K, Adachi K, Sasaki R, Monma S, Shioiri S, Seyama Y, et al. Randomized comparison of subcuticular sutures versus staples for skin closure after open abdominal surgery: a multicenter open-label randomized controlled trial. Journal of Gastrointestinal Surgery. 2016;20(12):2083–92.

32. Caballero Bermejo AF, Ruiz-Antorán B, Fernández Cruz A, Diago Sempere E, Callejas Díaz A, Múñez Rubio E, et al. Sarilumab versus standard of care for the early treatment of COVID-19 pneumonia in hospitalized patients: SARTRE: a structured summary of a study protocol for a randomised controlled trial. Trials. 2020;21(1):794.

33. Emens LA, Esteva FJ, Beresford M, Saura C, De Laurentiis M, Kim SB, et al. Trastuzumab emtansine plus atezolizumab versus trastuzumab emtansine plus placebo in previously treated, HER2-positive advanced breast cancer (KATE2): a phase 2, multicentre, randomised, double-blind trial. Lancet Oncology. 2020;21(10):1283–95.

34. Pocovi NC, Lin CC, Latimer J, Merom D, Tiedemann A, Maher C, et al. Effectiveness and cost-effectiveness of a progressive, individualised walking and education programme for prevention of low back pain recurrence in adults: study protocol for the WalkBack randomised controlled trial. BMJ Open. 2020;10(10):e037149.

35. Cremolini C, Antoniotti C, Rossini D, Lonardi S, Loupakis F, Pietrantonio F, et al. Upfront FOLFOXIRI plus bevacizumab and reintroduction after progression versus mFOLFOX6 plus bevacizumab followed by FOLFIRI plus bevacizumab in the treatment of patients with metastatic colorectal cancer (TRIBE2): a multicentre, open-label, phase 3, randomised, controlled trial. Lancet Oncology. 2020;21(4):497–507.

36. Thall PF, Wathen JK. Practical Bayesian adaptive randomisation in clinical trials. European Journal of Cancer. 2007;43(5):859–66.

37. Faderl S, Ravandi F, Huang X, Garcia-Manero G, Ferrajoli A, Estrov Z, et al. A randomized study of clofarabine versus clofarabine plus low-dose cytarabine as front-line therapy for patients aged 60 years and older with acute myeloid leukemia and high-risk myelodysplastic syndrome. Blood. 2008;112(5):1638–45.

38. Odutayo A, Emdin CA, Hsiao AJ, Shakir M, Copsey B, Dutton S, et al. Association between trial registration and positive study findings: cross sectional study (Epidemiological Study of Randomized Trials—ESORT). BMJ. 2017;356:j917.

39. Berger VW, Odia I. Characterizing permuted block randomization as a big stick procedure. Contemporary Clinical Trials Communications. 2016;2:80–4.

40. Weijer C, Enkin MW, Shapiro SH, Glass KC. Clinical equipoise and not the uncertainty principle is the moral underpinning of the randomised controlled trial—for & against. BMJ. 2000;321(7263):756.

4

Alternative randomized controlled trial designs

> [O]ne of America's brightest up-coming researchers was very frank,
> 'Bill,' she said, 'your trials are so boring!'
>
> **William Silverman, 2004 (1)**

Why use an alternative trial design?

In Chapter 3 we considered implicitly what might be called the standard RCT design. More formally we might describe it as a two-arm parallel group trial (Figure 4.1). Along with this design we typically are also conducting a trial which is 'definitive' in the sense that it seeks to provide an actionable finding without resort to further studies or evidence. Whether or not a single clinical trial is typically sufficient to achieve this is an interesting area for consideration but the key point here is that the study *seeks to provide an answer which could be acted upon*. In the language of study design this study might also be

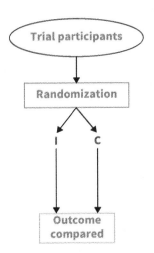

Standard RCT

- Features
  - Participants randomly allocated to one of two treatments
  - Fixed allocation ratio (typically even, i.e. 50/ 50 chance)
  - A single follow-up period identical in both arms
- Type of trial
  - Definitive study
  - Typically superiority question
  - Two-arm individually randomised parallel group design

Figure 4.1 Standard RCT design.

described as a phase 3 clinical trial. Some phase 2 clinical trials might also be considered somewhat definitive in the sense they confirm whether to proceed to a phase 3 clinical trial. Nevertheless, their clinical efficacy findings are considered provisional or preliminary, and in need of further confirmation in a phase 3 clinical trial. Note that there are a range of study designs under somewhat loose terms of feasibility and pilot studies which are not considered here. The use of some of the alternative designs covered in this chapter might form part of such a 'feasibility' assessment given the corresponding implications.

There are many variations on the standard RCT design which still involve randomization of treatments or other interventions. In this chapter we will consider some of the ways in which the design might be altered and some of the more common randomized trial designs. It is useful to consider why we might choose something other than the standard design. This is particularly important given it has been widely used and it is challenging enough to conduct any RCT as we will discuss further in Chapters 6–8. There are three main reasons why an alternative design might be chosen:

1. An alternative trial design might enable more than one research question to be addressed. As we saw in Chapter 2, there is a clear (or at least should be) link between the primary objective of a study and the design. The primary objective should in turn reflect the key research question which prompted the study. In some cases we may be able to address multiple related research questions in the same study if we alter the design. We clearly do not want to do this in a way which compromises how well we address the main research question of interest. However, if we can do so why should we not answer additional questions? Given that all clinical trials, and RCTs in particular, are very expensive, time-consuming, and demanding to conduct, if we could get more out of a single study it is certainly worth considering. Related to this, we may have two research questions which are equally relevant and a study answering either will not be sufficient to progress understanding substantially. Or put another way, there may be two relevant parts of a single overall question. For example, perhaps we have a new drug but two plausible dose levels with no apparent difference in safety even after previous early phase clinical trials. We clearly wish to know if the drug works, so it would intuitively be sensible to compare use of the drug against either the current clinical standard (which might be no treatment) or preferably (at least from a perspective of minimizing bias), a placebo control. However, we do not know which dose to select as there is a presumed trade-off between efficacy and the risk of adverse events. A design that allows us to deal with

the two possible dose levels without having to opt for one a priori as well as allowing a comparison against a control would be attractive.

2. An alternative design may be more efficient in some way. For example, it may require fewer participants to be recruited, it could be cheaper to run, or may be completed more quickly (e.g. as the sample size will be much lower). Any of these reasons on their own could justify the use of an alternative trial design.

3. In some circumstances the standard trial may not be practical or considered ethical which requires us to consider alternative designs. If there are three well-established treatment options, restricting treatment to two of these is difficult in terms of recruitment but arguably more fundamentally in terms of ethics. Alternatively, some element of the standard design when applied to the specific research question of interest, or the context in which the clinical trial will be conducted, may be very difficult to implement.

The standard design implies a number of things are possible which may not work for a specific context. The key one is that it requires recruitment of individuals and the ability to modify the treatment received by each individual. For some interventions which are already in clinical use, particularly, non-drug ones, it may be very difficult to achieve such control over the delivery in this way in a research study. For example, an education programme aimed at improving the prescribing of family doctors would naturally be applied to the family doctor, *not* the patient. It is therefore difficult, if not implausible, to expect the doctor to apply or not apply the training they have received depending upon an allocation given for the individual patient. Some interventions in the public health sphere may most naturally apply to a community or a geographical area, such as fluorination of water supply. It is not practical to vary this between households if they share the same water supply. Therefore, for a variety of reasons we may be forced to consider other designs as the standard one may be very difficult to implement.

A plethora of options

There are a very large, and ever-increasing, number of clinical trial designs. It is well beyond the scope of this book to cover even a substantial proportion of them in any detail, let alone all of them. For those uncomfortable with extensive mathematics this should come as a relief, as many differ in fairly subtle ways which require substantive consideration of the statistical aspects. This chapter will cover some of the more common ways in which trial designs can be altered from the standard RCT design. In turn, the following modifications will be considered: (i) varying the randomization options, (ii) varying what is randomized, (iii) using adaptive designs, and (iv) supra-trial designs. These are all summarized and considered relatively briefly but references to allow them and related topics to be studied in more detail have been provided for the interested reader.

Varying the randomization options

Multi-arm trial design

The most obvious and natural extension from a standard trial design is to have more than two randomization options (i.e. an RCT with more than two arms). Such a design is called a *multi-arm trial*. Moving from two to even just three treatment arms, surprisingly, can substantially increase the complexity in terms of design, conduct, analysis, and interpretation. A recent example is a trial treating patients with chronic rhinosinusitis who can undergo various treatments typically starting with intranasal medication (e.g. corticosteroid and saline irrigation) (2). Where symptoms are persistent and substantial, further treatments with antibiotics or nasal surgery are considerations. One option here would be to compare antibiotics and surgery in a two-arm (standard design) trial though the evidence for the use of both is uncertain. Therefore, a natural study to run would be one with a third treatment group (standard care, i.e. without the antibiotic or surgery). This latter treatment group could take different forms, for example, it could be standard care such as continuation of current treatment without an additional treatment, or continuation of current treatment with a placebo control. Either way, a three-arm trial could be seen as a much better (and valuable) study than a single two-arm trial and perhaps even better than two separate two-arm trials which may well differ in populations and important ways which can inhibit generalization (2). By including this third arm, participants are faced with a study where they might receive three quite different treatment options. The appropriate intervention and follow-up period similarly require careful thought.

As well as the practical impact for running the study, and patient and health professional participation, the increase in the number of trial arms from two makes a variety of statistical comparisons possible. In fact, we have seven possible ways to analyse the data from just three treatment groups. The possible options are shown in Figure 4.2 where we have intervention 1 (I_1), intervention 2 (I_2), and control treatment (C) groups. As the number of arms increase,

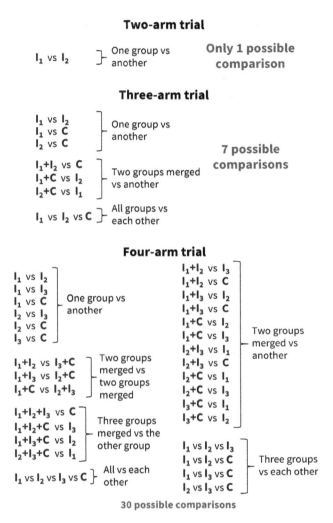

Figure 4.2 Possible statistical comparisons for two-, three-, and four-arm trials.

the potential number of comparisons that can be made escalates quickly (for four arms we have 30 different possibilities). These are again shown in Figure 4.2 which shows the options for four treatments—intervention 1 (I_1), intervention 2 (I_2), intervention 3 (I_3), and control treatment (C) groups. These comparison options relate to different, sometimes only subtly so, research questions. The main types of questions are (i) is there any difference between the groups (e.g. a comparison of all the groups simultaneously of which there is always only one such comparison); (ii) is there a difference between pairs of treatments (there are three ways to do this for a three-arm trial), and (iii) does one group differ from a combined group of the other groups (there are three ways to do this for a three-arm trial)? It is highly unlikely that we would be interested in all of these comparisons equally. Some are naturally secondary questions or related to others when the specific treatments to be evaluated are considered. While the comparison of all groups (e.g. I_1 versus I_2 versus control for a three-arm trial design) simultaneously may seem the most natural main comparison, it is not a sufficient place for the statistical analysis to finish. The reason for this is while identifying that all three treatments are not the same would be interesting (if we do observe this), it naturally begs the question which treatments differ from which, and by how much? Alternatively, if no difference overall is clearly identified, some quantification of the uncertain is needed and this will require further (pairwise) comparisons. Beyond the complexity of interpretation thrown up by multiple results we also have an underlying statistical concern to address. We need to limit our potential for misleading findings due to random chance. The more comparisons we do, the more likely we will observe chance findings. Both the appearance of differences when they do not truly exist, and also the occurrence of spuriously inconsistent findings are possible. Such a concern underlies two common steps in designing a clinical trial: (i) the choice of a primary outcome, and (ii) the determination of the sample size calculation based upon the primary outcome (see Chapters 2 and 5).

The key step in planning a multi-arm trial is to carefully consider the comparison options and their relative importance. It is critical that both the key research question and the primary objective of the study are kept in mind. No right answer exists and each situation needs to be considered in its own right. The value of comparing each treatment group depends upon our belief about how different each treatment group is. In the earlier rhinosinusitis example, all three treatment groups reflect quite distinct treatment options and therefore there is no a priori reason to expect some findings to be related. In contrast, if we have a six-arm trial where five arms have different dose regimens for the same active agent, and the other treatment aim is a placebo control, we are in a very different situation. In particular, it would be surprising if only one dose regimen were to be effective. Comparing all five dose regimens individually against the placebo control would substantially increase the potential for a chance finding (as we have five results). The analysis approach we adopt should match expectations about how the drug might work. An obvious approach would be to compare a combined group of all five dose regimens against the placebo group. A secondary comparison could explore differences between dose levels to ascertain a dose–response effect. This approach implies we think we roughly have the doses right but we are not sure which is optimal. This might be due to uncertainty about safety rather than the sufficiency of the dose levels to induce an effect in the primary outcome (should the drug actually work). The analysis strategy could be altered according to views on the potential dose levels (based upon, say, phase 1 and 2 clinical trials), and the sample size of the relative groups could be varied accordingly.

A potential benefit of multi-arm trials is the potential for more efficient trial designs. In this context 'efficiency' can mean various things (e.g. statistical efficiency). Crudely put, efficiency in trial design might be thought of as related to the number of participants needed overall, and the corresponding cost to run the trial. Two interesting variations of multi-arm trials are of particular note. First, a special type of multi-arm trial is called a factorial trial. In a factorial trial, the individual treatments and combinations of them are included as the randomization options. The treatments to be compared need to be combinable with each other and are referred to as 'factors' in this context; hence the name 'factorial trial' for RCTs with this type of design. For example, six interventions (all with only two levels, i.e. you receive it or you do not) to reduce nausea and vomiting after surgery were compared in a single RCT using a factorial design. This study allocated participants to one of the 64 (i.e. 2^6) possible combinations of the treatment factors(3). The design is efficient in that the sample size required is reduced compared to six separate trials, one for each intervention, if the factors (interventions) are thought to work independently. Under this scenario the impact of each intervention can be analysed separately as if the study is only looking at the respective factor. This is done by separating the participants into two groups, those who receive and those who do not receive the respective intervention. In the aforementioned example, the data can be analysed as if there were six separate trials, one for each factor (4 mg of ondansetron or none, 4 mg of dexamethasone or none, 1.25 mg of droperidol or none, propofol or a volatile anaesthetic, nitrogen or nitrous oxide, and remifentanil or fentanyl). However, if the factors do not work independently the interpretation is complication, and the analysis should really default to that of a typical multi-arm design (as a combination acts like different treatment options). As the number of combinations can get very large quickly, and some may be more challenging to deliver than others, sometimes only a subset of combinations will be allowed. A trial with this set-up is referred to as a partial factorial trial.

Second, a multi-arm design also allows for the potential of multiple assessments and therefore the potential to vary the treatments under evaluation during the course of running the study. Such an approach naturally facilitates adaptive designs which we will consider later in this chapter. Adoption of either of these special cases (factorial or adaptive multi-arm designs) has implications for the sample size, conduct, and analysis of the study (4,5).

Varying what is randomized

Under an alternative trial design we can vary what is randomized. Typically in clinical trials we are randomizing individuals to receive a particular treatment, and that individual is usually, though not always, a patient. However, this does not need to be the case and different trial designs have been proposed which randomize different units. Broadly, these fall into four options regarding what is randomized:

- Parts of the body (e.g. the left knee to the intervention, the right knee to the control).
- Sequential periods of different treatments on the same individual (e.g. treatment with the intervention drug followed by treatment with the control drug or vice versa).
- Receipt of a single treatment (e.g. intervention drug versus control drug as per a standard RCT design), or
- Randomizing groups of individuals to a treatment (e.g. all the patients under the care of the same family doctor receive either the intervention or the control).

Table 4.1 gives a summary of the options and a corresponding trial design with an example trial which uses this design. For all of these designs it is possible (in principle) to vary the number of treatment arms and indeed combine elements. Mostly these designs are utilized with only two treatment groups. However, there is nothing in principle precluding the use of multi-arms in combination with randomization of the different possible units. Indeed, some of these modifications can be used together (e.g. a cluster crossover design) (6). As each of the options leads to different alternative trial designs, we will briefly consider these in turn.

Table 4.1 Different randomization options

Unit of randomization	Examples of unit	Trial design	Trial example
Part of the body to a single treatment	Knee, arm, leg, area of skin, eye, etc.	Within-person trial	Comparison of two surgical approaches (subvastus and midvastus) to carrying out a total knee arthroplasty (7) Participants with bilateral osteoarthritis were randomized to receive the subvastus operation on their right or left knee and the midvastus approach on the other knee
Sequential treatment periods on the same individual	A 12-week treatment period	Crossover trial	Comparison of morphine or methadone maintenance programme for people dependent on opioids (8). Each participant was allocated to receive methadone oral solution for 11 weeks (1 adjustment plus 10 treatment weeks) followed by slow-release oral morphine for the same period or vice versa. A 2 × 2 crossover trial design
A single treatment received by an individual	Patient, healthy volunteer	Individually randomized parallel group trial (i.e. standard design when there are only two arms)	Comparison of pertuzumab, trastuzumab, and docetaxel versus placebo, trastuzumab, and docetaxel in patients with HER2-postive metastatic breast cancer (9)
Group of individuals ('cluster') who receive the same single treatment	Household, patients under care of a health professional, hospital, community	Cluster trial	Comparison of bendiocarb indoor residual spraying or deltamethrin indoor residual spraying difference in terms of malaria control (10); 24 geographical areas (minimum of 250 households) in central Malabo on Bioko Island, Equatorial Guinea, were allocated to receive bendiocarb or deltamethrin indoor residual spraying

Within-person trial design

The within-person design refers to studies where the random allocation of treatment is to multiple units (such as body parts or organs) per participant. In the example in Table 4.1, it is two knees per participant which are allocated to one or the other of the two treatments under evaluation (in this case two surgical operations). Most commonly the within-person design has been used to assess two treatments on limbs, or on organs which most people have two of, such as eyes. The design has been used to assess treatments upon organs (e.g. eyes), and other body parts (e.g. areas of skin). However, even where more than two units could be evaluated, often only two units per individual are used (e.g. in 'spilt-mouth' designs in dentistry, instead of assessing individual teeth the mouth is typically divided into two parts). This is presumably for simplicity of application and interpretation of findings. The main attraction of using a within-person design is that it is statistically more efficient than a standard design (which in contrast is sometimes referred to as a 'between-person' design, reflecting the data used in the analysis). It is not difficult to understand why a within-person trial design can be advantageous. In this design, the participant's outcome after treatment of one unit is compared to the *same* participant's outcome after treatment of another unit. The treatments are therefore compared using data from the same individual, thus removing variability due to differences between individuals (i.e. due to age, ethnicity, biological sex, genetics, social factors, etc.).

There are a number of key features about a within-person design which should be noted. First, the treatments to be randomized need to be deliverable at the within-person (i.e. unit) level. For example, eye drops can clearly be given to each eye individually and therefore each eye can be treated differently. However, a systemic medicine given orally, such as an antibiotic for an eye infection like conjunctivitis, clearly cannot. Second, in addition to a treatment that can be delivered at the within-person level, at least some key outcomes need to be assessable for the unit. Preferably the outcome of one unit is completely unaffected by the treatment of any other unit on the same person. Some outcomes may not be clearly assessable separately for each unit (e.g. mortality). For the knee surgery example, the two operations were conducted sequentially on different days with a gap of 8–12 weeks between them. Some outcomes could clearly be assessed separately for each treatment (e.g. operation time, operative complications, and radiographic knee-specific assessments). Others such as walking and generally mobility clearly cannot as the benefit of surgery on one knee influences the individual's overall mobility. Most difficult to deal with are some outcomes which fall in a middle group where they can be assessed at the knee level (such as assessing postoperative pain for each knee) but the outcome will likely be influenced by the treatment of the other knee. The impact of one treatment upon another in this context has been described as a 'carry-across' effect. This makes both interpretation and potentially the statistical analysis more difficult. An important distinction should be made between studies where the within-person units are treated concurrently or sequentially (as in the knee surgery example).

Third, the use of a within-person design requires the sample size to be determined in a way that takes into account the use of multiple outcomes per participant. These outcomes are no longer independent and thus this needs to be recognized accordingly. Where there are only two units per participant, these types of data are often referred to in statistical literature as 'paired' data. For a continuous outcome such data can be analysed with a paired t-test and a corresponding sample size calculation should be used. Relative to a corresponding standard design (e.g. same anticipated population, same outcome and target difference, etc.), the sample size is substantially reduced in a within-person design. Initially it might be thought the required sample size is one-half (for a within-person study of two treatments with two units per person). In fact, it can be substantially less than this. How much so depends upon the degrees of similarity in outcome between sites within the same person. In the simplest case, the relationship between the sample size required in a within-person design with two units and a standard (1:1 parallel-group) design can be estimated for a continuous outcome (making the assumption of normality) as follows:

$$N_{within-person} = \frac{(1-\rho)N_{parallel-group}}{2}$$

where ρ is what is called the Pearson correlation between the outcome at the two units for each participant (11). This correlation varies between 0 and 1 with a value of 0 indicating no relationship between outcomes for the same person (i.e. it is no more similar than random chance). A value of 1 indicates complete agreement in outcome (though not necessarily identical values). The greater this correlation, the greater the reduction in sample size needed for a within-person trial. In Chapter 5 we will consider how to calculate sample size calculations for a standard trial design. To show the potential impact of the use of a within-person design we use an example where the standard (parallel-group) design requires 100 participants overall (50 per group). If correlation for the outcome was relatively low (0.2), we can see that only $\frac{0.8 \times 100}{2} = 40$ participants (less than half) are required for the within-person design. If the correlation were moderately high (0.5), only $\frac{0.5 \times 100}{2} = 25$ participants are required (i.e. one-quarter of the number of a corresponding parallel group trial). The same simple formula above works reasonably well as an approximation for a binary outcome where the final estimated sample size (after the reduction for the within-person design) is still a reasonable size (such as 50 or more). A more precise calculation can be produced based upon McNemar's test (12).

Fourth, to correspond with the modified sample size, the statistical analysis should account for the similarity of outcomes for units within the same person. In the simplest case of two units per participant, a paired t-test could be used for a continuous outcome, and for a binary outcome the paired difference in proportions could be calculated with an appropriate confidence interval method (13). Where there are more than two units per person, more complex methods such as generalized estimating equations or multilevel models can be used (11). Time-to-event outcomes are more difficult to analyse as standard methods are not appropriate (14). Whatever the outcome of interest, the analysis may also need to consider the possibility of a carry-across effect. Fifth, the reporting of such a trial is subtly different from a standard trial design and this will be considered further in Chapter 10.

Crossover trial design

In a crossover trial, instead of allocating participants to a single treatment and follow-up period, they are allocated to a sequence of treatments with data collected for each period in the sequence. In the simplest form, there are two treatments (intervention and control) and two time periods (a 2 × 2 crossover trial design). The possible allocations for this design are then simply IC and CI; that is, allocation to the intervention treatment during time period 1 and the control treatment during time period 2, or vice versa. Figure 4.3 shows visually the key difference between the standard design and a 2 × 2 crossover design. The letters indicate the treatments in the possible allocations and the arrows indicate the follow-up. In the standard design, participants are

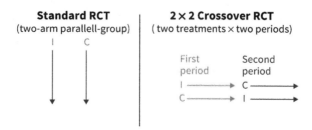

Figure 4.3 Standard versus crossover trial designs.

allocated to I or C and do not change treatment. In the crossover trial, they are allocated to the sequence IC or CI. Such a design is sometimes referred to as the 'AB/BA' crossover design given these only (two) possible treatment sequences (here we have used I and C instead of A and B for consistency with previous examples).

In the example given in Table 4.1, the allocation is to receive morphine for 11 weeks followed by methadone for 11 weeks, or 11 weeks of methadone followed by 11 weeks of morphine. Similar to a within-person trial design, the key benefit is that each participant acts as their own control. However, the crossover trial differs from the within-person design in that the whole person receives the same allocation. Additional treatments are always received sequentially. In the following discussion, it will generally be assumed that a comparison of only two treatments is in mind and that the two time-period (2 × 2) design is in mind though it should be noted there is no reason (other than simplicity) that such a design is used. There are potential advantages in terms of the sample size and statistical analysis from using more elaborate designs provided they can be implemented (15).

The key assumption of a crossover trial is the ability of the participant to return to, in essence, their original state prior to the commencement of the second (and any further) time period. If the outcome at the start of subsequent periods is affected by the treatment(s) which precedes it, this undermines the value of the design. Such an occurrence is called a 'carry-over' effect. Accordingly, a crossover design tends to be used for relatively 'stable' and chronic conditions such as treatment for liver disease. It is an odd design to use when the main outcome of interest is a critical event (e.g. pregnancy when treating for infertility) which cannot realistically occur in multiple time period (16). To facilitate the return to a 'typical' state, it is common to have a 'washout' period, that is, a time gap between the formal time periods during which the treatments are given and the outcome is measured. This period needs to be long enough for any effect of the preceding treatment's effect to have waned. The term 'washout' come from the typical use of the design to compare two drug interventions. A washout period of 7–14 days between treatment periods is common though the length will need to vary according to the treatments being evaluated. Interestingly, in the crossover trial of treatment for people dependent on opioids described in Table 4.1, there was no gap between the treatments but instead there was a 1-week period during which the treatment was received and for which outcome was not measured. Understandably, any absence of treatment was thought to likely lead to substantial withdrawal of participants from the study. The hope is that the status at the start of the second period can in essence be considered to be the same as the original one when the participant entered the first treatment period study. If this is the case, we get multiple results from each participant with the additional benefit of having the result on the same set of individuals. This statistical efficiency is reflected in the sample size required in contrast to a corresponding parallel group trial. However, if the status of the second period is not the same as the first period, we have what is called a 'period effect'. This complicates the statistical analysis and interpretation of findings.

Relative to a parallel group trial the efficiency gain of using a 2 × 2 cross-over design for an outcome (making the typical assumption of normality for the outcome data) can be calculated using the same formula given above for a within-person trial. The only difference is that here ρ represents the correlation between the outcome measured for the same person at the two time periods and not two units within a person. For example, a parallel group trial seeking to detect a 10 mmHg difference in systolic blood pressure with 15 mmHg standard deviation with two-sided significance level of 5% and 80% statistical power would require 74 (37 per group) participants. If the correlation between outcomes is assumed to be 0.5, then using a 2 × 2 crossover trial would lead a sample size one-quarter of the size of the standard trial design. In this case this is just 19 participants. The reduction in the number of participants is very sensitive to the assumed correlation value. Were it to be as high as 0.8 then the sample size required is one-tenth of that of a standard trial. It is worth noting that the variance of interest in the crossover trial is not the same as the parallel group trial. In the crossover trial we are interested in the within-person variability whereas in a parallel group trial it is the between-person variability. This latter quantity is much larger as it is calculated from measurements on different people rather than for two measurements on the same person. While in principle the above sample size adjustment for within-person trials generally applies also to a binary outcome, it is not generally useful for crossover trials as these tend to have very small samples sizes (<30 participants) (17). A calculation based upon McNemar's test is more appropriate for a binary outcome (12). Sample size calculations can become quite elaborate where greater numbers of treatment and time period are involved, particularly so if the evaluating period or carry-over effect is of interest. More extensive consideration of the analysis of crossover trials is given elsewhere (15).

Another feature of a crossover trial is that they have multiple follow-up periods and therefore will take longer to run (for the same length of follow-up) than a standard design. Accordingly, the crossover design tends to be used to assess for relatively short-term outcomes (e.g. weeks rather than months or years). Related to the benefit of its efficiency is the more problematic nature of any missing observation (as each observation contributes more data).

Unfortunately, if we do not have the result for a participant for one time period, we cannot readily use their data. Therefore, the loss per piece of data is more problematic than a parallel group trial. The statistical analysis of a crossover trial can also be more complicated compared to a standard trial design. If there is a systematic difference between the treatment effect measured in the different time periods, the statistical analysis and interpretation is complicated. There are two different broad possibilities that may occur. First, treatment in later period(s) may differ systematically from the first period as noted above ('period effect'). This could be due to individuals tending towards better or worse outcome over time (e.g. regression to the mean). Or another possibility is something external to the trial may have changed the underlying healthcare which in turn affects the outcome of patients in the later time period(s), for example, implementation of a new treatment protocol for all patients. Second, there could be a period-by-treatment interaction effect (i.e. the treatments work differently in the different period). This is the worst situation to be in. The most likely reason for this is that the effect of the treatment carries over into the subsequent period, a 'carry-over' effect. However, it could be due to another cause other than a residual treatment effect from the previous time period. Unfortunately, the very efficiency of a crossover trial in its simplest form makes teasing out of these possibilities in the statistical analysis very difficult. A period effect, where the treatment effect under one period differs from the other (the first possibility we considered above), is a much more tractable problem (15,16). More complex crossover designs (e.g. three or more treatment periods per participant) can be used to allow exploration of such effects. However, this is at the cost of increasing complexity in study delivery, and the potential for a reduction in the length of follow-up per period.

As with the within-person design, statistical analysis approaches that take into account the paired nature of the data are needed. Simpler analysis options include paired t-tests for a continuous outcome. Correspondingly, a McNemar test and confidence intervals for paired proportions or an odds ratio for a binary outcome could be used. The crossover design does not naturally suit a time-to-event-based analysis unless events can occur more than once, and therefore we do not consider this further.

Cluster trial

In a cluster randomized trial (hereafter simply called a cluster trial), a group of individuals are randomly allocated to receive a treatment instead of being allocated individually (18). An example is shown in Figure 4.4 where six clusters

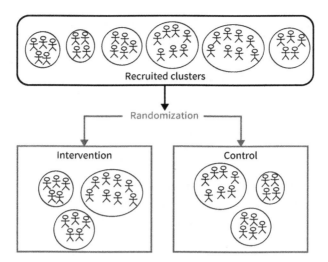

Figure 4.4 Cluster randomized trial example with six clusters.

are allocated into either the intervention or the control group. The cluster trial design is more commonly used for non-drug interventions; the design is not used in a regulatory drug evaluation setting.

The sample size required for a cluster trial, unlike a crossover or within-person design, will be larger than that required for a standard (parallel group) design trial. The relative difference can be approximated for a continuous or binary outcome using this formula:

$$1 + \left(\bar{n}_{cluster} - 1\right) ICC$$

where $\bar{n}_{cluster}$ is the average cluster size expected and ICC is the intracluster correlation. The ICC is a measure of how much of the overall variance can be attributed to the cluster an individual belongs to. This sample size adjustment presumes a statistical analysis which uses the individual participant's data (as opposed to only using cluster level summaries). The size of the ICC will vary depending on a number of factors. Collections of ICC estimates calculated from previous studies have been produced to aid determination of appropriate sample sizes (19). Relatively small ICC values can lead to substantial increases in the sample size. For example, if the cluster size is 50, an ICC of only 0.02 will lead to almost a doubling of the sample size required. The magnitude of this loss can be offset by having more clusters of a smaller size. If we had a cluster size of only 10, then an ICC of only 0.11 would double the required sample. The ideal situation would be a cluster trial with large number of small clusters.

However, typically there is limited flexibility around the number and size of clusters in practice (e.g. there are only a limited number of teaching hospitals in a country). Fortunately, as the cluster size increases, the ICC tends to decrease though it is quite possible a cluster trial is not a practical option for a specific research question due to the required sample size. There is a clear disadvantage in terms of the number of observations using a cluster trial, and the implications of this need careful consideration at the outset (20). Where the cluster size is anticipated to vary substantially, the sample size calculation can be adjusted accordingly to account for this, which leads to a (even) larger overall sample size (21).

Given this clear disadvantage in terms of the overall sample size, why would one use a cluster trial design? There are a number of possible reasons. A cluster randomized trial may be the only realistic way to deliver the study. A parallel group trial design requires manipulation of the treatment received between each participant. However, in many settings this is implausible, or at least burdensome. For example, if we are assessing a community level intervention, such as in our cluster randomization example in Table 4.1, the practicalities of varying application between households are very difficult to implement at the scale which is likely to be required to observe a sufficient number of events. An educational intervention which involves providing information to some within a cluster may lead to others receiving, even if in a somewhat lessor or diluted way, the intervention. For example, health professional-focused educational interventions (e.g. prescribing of antibiotics) may lead to sharing of information between colleagues who work together. The potential for the intervention to be received by those for whom it is not intended has been referred to in this context as a 'contamination' effect. It has the potential to dilute any difference between the intervention and control groups. Other interventions may naturally involve a group and therefore naturally fit a cluster trial design. For example, one intervention seeking to influence the prescribing practice of family doctors will impact all of the relevant patients under the care of that doctor.

There are a number of key features of cluster trials to note:

1. As the cluster is to be randomized, the intervention and control need to be applicable to the whole of each cluster. An intervention like surgery will not typically work in this way given capacity constraints upon surgeons, operating theatres, and so on. That is before we consider whether any surgeons would be willing to accept such a loss of control over the treatment of patients. On the other hand, group therapy, IT-based interventions, and public health interventions might more readily be implemented in a cluster trial.

2. The ethical considerations of a cluster trial are of a different nature from a standard trial (22). Typically, some permission to apply an intervention to a cluster will be required (e.g. hospital management). However, this may be quite removed from those who receive the intervention or control (e.g. patients or healthcare professionals) and possibly also from whom the outcome data are collected for (e.g. patients). In some scenarios, consent of individual participants, and for the clusters involved is clearly necessary. In other scenarios, consent relating only to the clusters' involvement may be sufficient. The nature of the intervention, the implications of the trial for the individuals within the clusters, and the data to be collected are key points to consider.

3. As the number of clusters available to randomize is typically quite small, and the size of the clusters usually vary, some form of restricted randomization is typically used to help ensure balance on key cluster characteristics (e.g. size, and other factors strongly associated with outcome). Figure 4.4 shows the potential problem with only six clusters of unequal size leading to 16 and 18 individuals in the respective treatment groups. Had the allocation of clusters been different we could have had the two largest clusters in the sample group leading to a potential imbalance of 20 and 14 individuals in the treatment groups. In the example malaria trial in Table 4.1, the clusters were geographical areas chosen to have similar numbers of households within them. The randomization of the clusters controlled for the baseline prevalence of the disease, the number of households with nets, the proportion wanting indoor residual spraying, and the proportion who had used indoor residual spraying previously. All of these factors might reasonably predict the likelihood of a 2–14-year-old getting malaria.

4. Data collection also requires more careful consideration. In particular, care is needed to avoid bias when outcomes within clusters are collected. Those who contribute data in one cluster could differ somewhat from one another. In particular, cluster trials of interventions received at the individual level (e.g. physiotherapy given to individual patients where the hospital is allocated) are more susceptible to bias (23). If this occurs systematically between intervention and control groups it will lead to a bias in the observed effect. A related point is that the individuals within a cluster may change over time (e.g. patients are admitted or discharged from hospital during the follow-up period). The collection of data can be more complex and may require more assessments over time, or more proactive systems.

5. Lastly, cluster trials differ in terms of the statistical analysis. Unlike the previous trials there is no default level per se upon which to compare the intervention and control group data. We could compare data between the clusters, that is, what was randomized, and in some regards this is the obvious thing to do. However, we may be more interested in the outcome of the individuals within the clusters, and particularly so if the intervention and control are applied at the individual level (e.g. physiotherapy). Both strategies are potentially viable. If we analyse at the cluster level, we can proceed with a standard trial analysis but with the clusters being the unit of analysis. The caveat is that each observation is a summary for the relevant cluster, and that the number of observations in the number of clusters could be very small. Alternatively, if we analyse the data at the individual level, we need to use statistical analysis methods which account for the cluster to which each individual belongs. This is needed in order to get an appropriate estimation of the variation and the corresponding statistical uncertainty. Methods such as a multilevel or linear mixed model can be used to do this. Whichever approach is adopted our statistical analysis will need to be tailored accordingly to take into account the cluster design (24).

Adaptive versus fixed designs

The designs we have considered so far have been what might be termed as 'fixed' designs, that is, the study design is selected, the sample size required is determined, and the study is conducted according to the plan with the data analysed at the end of recruitment and follow-up. Implicitly no substantive changes are anticipated during the conduct of the study. However, this ignores the accumulating data which could help us refine the initial study design. Accordingly, designs which 'adapt' or are 'flexible' have been proposed which make use of available accumulating data in some way. A key point to note is that these are adaptive *designs*, that is, it is part of the design of the study (and addressed in the study protocol) from the outset that the design may adapt in this way. Furthermore, the type of adaptation, and, generally speaking, the rules by which we decide if such changes may take place, are determined in advance. Most notably, but by no means exclusively, such an adaptation will typically affect the trial's planned sample size. There is no longer a single sample size number of interest but various possibilities reflecting different scenarios that might occur. Accordingly, the statistical analysis may well need to be altered to include some formal statistical assessment to determine whether any adaption should take place at some point during the running of the study. Any such changes will obviously also have an impact upon all aspects of the study, some adaptations more than others. The aim is to have a study design which can address the uncertainty regarding one or more aspects of trial design in a way which may be more efficient and potentially provide more useful findings (5).

There are a very large number of potential aspects of a clinical trial which could be adapted as a trial progresses, but the more common aspects are as follows:

- Stopping the study early either for success or failure (in statistical terms due to 'efficacy' or 'futility' considerations respectively) (25).
- Altering the sample size (26).
- Changing the randomization treatment options (including the number and nature of the treatment options) (27).
- Identifying the most appropriate patients and altering eligibility (28).

These adaptations can all be applied to an individual clinical trial (e.g. any multi-arm trial). However, they often they go hand in hand with the conduct of multiple studies together (a 'supra-trial designs') which we will consider in more detail below. Either way the decision to make or not make a change to the ongoing trial is determined by the use in some way of interim data as part of a formal analysis. If well designed, any change, made according to the plan, will not undermine the validity of the study. This careful design is critical to ensure credibility of the findings and particularly where the trial may form part of a regulatory submission for approval of a drug for clinical use. As such, studies with adaptive designs tend to involve much more time spent prior to conduct focusing upon the statistical and practical implications of the design. Both the sample size and statistical analysis will need to be considered carefully to cover all the potential scenarios envisioned. In Chapter 7 we will consider formal statistical interim analyses which are typically used to determine whether an adaption should be made to the trial design.

Conducting many trials within a single study (supra-trial designs)

Often considered in conjunction with using an adaptive design, though strictly speaking a separate issue, is the use of a supra-trial design. This is a study which in essence contains multiple clinical trials within it. Various names have been used for different forms of this approach including 'platform'

(29), 'multi-arm multi-stage' (MAMS) (27), 'trials within cohorts' (TWiCs) (30), and 'basket' and 'umbrella' trials (31) to describe variations on the same theme. The distinction between the designs indicated by these terms can be quite subtle; platform and TWiCs emphasize the underlying study system upon which the individual studies are conducted. MAMS refers to the use of a multi-arm design with multiple stages at which the design of the study may change according to a planned analysis. A visual summary of the difference between basket, umbrella, and platform trials is given in Figure 4.5. Basket and umbrella designs refer to the inclusion of multiple diseases and multiple subpopulations respectively within a single study with a corresponding formal assessment of the treatment in conjunction with patient characteristics or biomarkers (31). In the drug regulatory setting there are also so-called seamless designs where are in essence two clinical trials run in the same study. For example, a seamless phase 1/2 trial design has been proposed where the phase 1 proportion is conducted (using a standard 3 + 3 dose escalation design) and

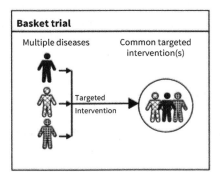
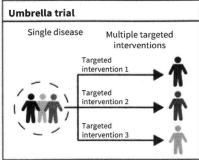
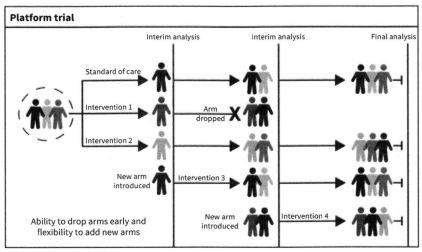

Figure 4.5 Basket, umbrella, and platform trials (31).

a phase 2 proportion using a selection design which seeks to identify the optimal dose according to both safety and efficacy (32). Different patients are recruited to the corresponding parts of the trial. The overall sample size and cost of running the study are potentially lower than if two separate clinical trials were conducted. Variations on this general approach exist though it is unclear how commonly seamless designs are used in practice.

Clearly, such supra-trial designs as considered above will not be appropriate for all situations. It is worth emphasizing that some of these trials are massive undertakings to deliver. While the statistical aspects have received the most attention within the scientific literature, the implications for trial management and coordination can be profound. Nevertheless, where used appropriately, they are very attractive and their use is becoming more common, though far from typical. In particular, the conduct of trials such as RECOVERY (Randomized Evaluation of Covid-19 Therapy) in the UK (29) and ACTT (Adaptive Covid-19 Treatment Trial) in the US (33) to address the treatment of COVID-19 has particularly highlighted the value (and need) for adaptive trials in providing quick (compared to usual) and relevant clinically findings. A key driver of their success has been the coordination across trial groups and with funders, and the support of the medical community.

How to decide which design to use

Given the somewhat bewildering array of trial designs and minor variations which grows year by year, even the most seasoned researcher might feel somewhat daunted at choosing a trial design. A few broad considerations need to be borne in mind. First, there is no single 'right' design, a number will be likely be fine with varying pros and cons. Some designs will be wrong in this instance for one or more reasons (such as timing, funding, interpretation, expertise required to deliver it, and impracticality of recruitment, among other considerations). Second, a trial that cannot be delivered is not a good one no matter how elegant its conception and statistical attributes. Implications of a design in terms of its running, timescale, and personnel need to be careful mulled over. Third, the standard design is the most common as it works, is relatively straightforward to apply, and has an obvious and clear interpretation. Some clear additional benefit should be required to move away from this design. Fourth, all trials are hard work to deliver, and place a burden upon participants. Therefore, the scope for improved efficiency, reduced burden on participants, and more relevant findings from using an alternative design should be carefully considered. Fifth, just as the tail should not wag the dog, the design should not determine the research questions, nor the hierarchy of them. Some designs naturally lead to addressing a particular type of research question. The real research questions of interest need to be kept in mind as the various trial designs, and what they can provide, are considered.

Summary

A range of alternative clinical trial designs are available which might suit particular research questions and settings. They can enable multiple research questions to be answered in a single study, or may be more practical than a standard trial design to conduct. Randomization can also be carried out in a different way from a standard clinical trial design. Each alternative design has its own advantages and disadvantages which need to be considered before a specific design can be chosen to address the research questions of interest. Given how time-consuming and expensive clinical trials are to carry out, the potential value of an alternative trial design should be considered. However, the corresponding impact upon trial conduct and related challenges need to be weighted up as well.

References

1. Silverman WA. Personal reflections on lessons learned from randomized trials involving newborn infants from 1951 to 1967. Clinical Trials. 2004;1(2):179–84.
2. Blackshaw H, Vennik J, Philpott C, Thomas M, Eyles C, Carpenter J, et al. Expert panel process to optimise the design of a randomised controlled trial in chronic rhinosinusitis (the MACRO programme). Trials. 2019;20(1):230.
3. Apfel CC, Korttila K, Abdalla M, Kerger H, Turan A, Vedder I, et al. A factorial trial of six interventions for the prevention of postoperative nausea and vomiting. New England Journal of Medicine. 2004;350(24):2441–51.
4. Montgomery AA, Peters TJ, Little P. Design, analysis and presentation of factorial randomised controlled trials. BMC Medical Research Methodology. 2003;3(1):26.
5. Pallmann P, Bedding AW, Choodari-Oskooei B, Dimairo M, Flight L, Hampson LV, et al. Adaptive designs in clinical trials: why use them, and how to run and report them. BMC Medicine. 2018;16(1):29.
6. Hooper R, Bourke L. Cluster randomised trials with repeated cross sections: alternatives to parallel group designs. BMJ. 2015;350:h2925.
7. Masjudin T, Kamari Z. A comparison between subvastus and midvastus approaches for staged bilateral total knee arthroplasty: a prospective, randomised study. Malaysian Orthopaedic Journal. 2012;6(3):31–6.
8. Beck T, Haasen C, Verthein U, Walcher S, Schuler C, Backmund M, et al. Maintenance treatment for opioid dependence with slow-release oral morphine: a randomized cross-over, non-inferiority study versus methadone. Addiction. 2014;109(4):617–26.

9. Swain SM, Kim SB, Cortés J, Ro J, Semiglazov V, Campone M, et al. Pertuzumab, trastuzumab, and docetaxel for HER2-positive metastatic breast cancer (CLEOPATRA study): overall survival results from a randomised, double-blind, placebo-controlled, phase 3 study. Lancet Oncology. 2013;14(6):461–71.

10. Bradley J, Hergott D, Garcia G, Lines J, Cook J, Slotman MA, et al. A cluster randomized trial comparing deltamethrin and bendiocarb as insecticides for indoor residual spraying to control malaria on Bioko Island, Equatorial Guinea. Malaria Journal. 2016;15(1):378.

11. Pandis N, Walsh T, Polychronopoulou A, Katsaros C, Eliades T. Split-mouth designs in orthodontics: an overview with applications to orthodontic clinical trials. European Journal of Orthodontics. 2013;35(6):783–9.

12. Obuchowski NA. Sample size calculations in studies of test accuracy. Statistical Methods in Medical Research. 1998;7(4):371–92.

13. Newcombe RG. Improved confidence intervals for the difference between binomial proportions based on paired data. Statistics in Medicine. 1998;17(22):2635–50.

14. Lesaffre E, Garcia Zattera MJ, Redmond C, Huber H, Needleman I. Reported methodological quality of split-mouth studies. Journal of Clinical Periodontology. 2007;34(9):756–61.

15. Senn S. Cross-Over Trials in Clinical Research. 2nd ed. Chichester: Wiley; 2002.

16. Elbourne DR, Altman DG, Higgins JP, Curtin F, Worthington HV, Vail A. Meta-analyses involving cross-over trials: methodological issues. International Journal of Epidemiology. 2002;31(1):140–9.

17. Mills EJ, Chan AW, Wu P, Vail A, Guyatt GH, Altman DG. Design, analysis, and presentation of crossover trials. Trials. 2009;10:27.

18. Campbell MJ, Walters SJ. How to Design, Analyse and Report Cluster Randomised Trials in Medicine and Health Related Research. Chichester: Wiley; 2014.

19. Cook JA, Bruckner T, MacLennan GS, Seiler CM. Clustering in surgical trials—database of intracluster correlations. Trials. 2012;13(1):2.

20. Hemming K, Eldridge S, Forbes G, Weijer C, Taljaard M. How to design efficient cluster randomised trials. BMJ. 2017;358:j3064.

21. Rutterford C, Copas A, Eldridge S. Methods for sample size determination in cluster randomized trials. International Journal of Epidemiology. 2015;44(3):1051–67.

22. Weijer C, Enkin MW, Shapiro SH, Glass KC. Clinical equipoise and not the uncertainty principle is the moral underpinning of the randomised controlled trial—for & against. BMJ. 2000;321(7263):756.

23. Easter C, Thompson JA, Eldridge S, Taljaard M, Hemming K. Cluster randomized trials of individual-level interventions were at high risk of bias. Journal of Clinical Epidemiology. 2021;138:49–59.

24. Eldridge S, Ukoumunne OC. A Practical Guide to Cluster Randomised Trials in Health Services Research. Oxford: Wiley; 2012.

25. Snapinn S, Chen MG, Jiang Q, Koutsoukos T. Assessment of futility in clinical trials. Pharmaceutical Statistics. 2006;5(4):273–81.

26. Kolias AG, Edlmann E, Thelin EP, Bulters D, Holton P, Suttner N, et al. Dexamethasone for adult patients with a symptomatic chronic subdural haematoma (Dex-CSDH) trial: study protocol for a randomised controlled trial. Trials. 2018;19(1):670.

27. James ND, Sydes MR, Mason MD, Clarke NW, Anderson J, Dearnaley DP, et al. Celecoxib plus hormone therapy versus hormone therapy alone for hormone-sensitive prostate cancer: first results from the STAMPEDE multiarm, multistage, randomised controlled trial. Lancet Oncology. 2012;13(5):549–58.

28. Mittendorf EA, Zhang H, Barrios CH, Saji S, Jung KH, Hegg R, et al. Neoadjuvant atezolizumab in combination with sequential nab-paclitaxel and anthracycline-based chemotherapy versus placebo and chemotherapy in patients with early-stage

triple-negative breast cancer (IMpassion031): a randomised, double-blind, phase 3 trial. Lancet. 2020;396(10257):1090–100.

29. Recovery Collaborative Group. Dexamethasone in hospitalized patients with Covid-19. New England Journal of Medicine. 2020;384(8):693–704.

30. Gal R, Monninkhof EM, van Gils CH, Groenwold RHH, Elias SG, van den Bongard D, et al. Effects of exercise in breast cancer patients: implications of the trials within cohorts (TwiCs) design in the UMBRELLA Fit trial. Breast Cancer Research and Treatment. 2021;190(1):89–101.

31. Park JJH, Siden E, Zoratti MJ, Dron L, Harari O, Singer J, et al. Systematic review of basket trials, umbrella trials, and platform trials: a landscape analysis of master protocols. Trials. 2019;20(1):572.

32. Hoering A, LeBlanc M, Crowley J. Seamless phase I–II trial design for assessing toxicity and efficacy for targeted agents. Clinical Cancer Research. 2011;17(4):640–6.

33. Beigel JH, Tomashek KM, Dodd LE, Mehta AK, Zingman BS, Kalil AC, et al. Remdesivir for the treatment of Covid-19—final report. New England Journal of Medicine. 2020;383(19):1813–26.

5

Choosing the sample size for a clinical trial

> In short, there is, and can be, no magic number for either clinician or statistician.
>
> **Bradford Hill, 1952 (1)**

Choosing the sample size

Determining an appropriate sample size is perhaps the most critical aspect of designing a clinical trial after defining the research question. It has a huge impact on all aspects of the study. While the justification for a chosen sample size is typically a statistical one, the sample size will clearly have an operational impact on the study and whether it is actually deliverable. For example, moving from a study of 20 participants to one of 200 participants may well require multiple study centres. At the very least, it will require more recruitment time per centre, and additional funding to support the larger sample size. Having more than one study centre has other implications, such as having sufficient resources so that each centre can accommodate the study requirements and processes. It may also require greater flexibility in the study's overall approach. All research studies including clinical trials operate within certain financial and practical constraints, such as the personnel available (both study team members and centre staff) and who is in the population of interest. A statistical justification for the sample size, although of great value, is not the sole determinant of the sample size.

More fundamentally, we have an ethical imperative to ensure that the study being carried out is one that will likely answer the main research question. We are asking people to take part in a study that could expose them to risks they may not otherwise be exposed to. At the very least, we are asking them to bear a burden in terms of research-associated activities, such as extra visits to a hospital, receiving medical tests, completing forms about their health, and collecting medical data on them. These risks and burdens can only be ethically justifiable if the study has a chance of providing useful insights. Getting the sample size right is absolutely key to giving the study the chance of making a real difference to what we currently know.

The first step is to formulate the clinical trial's objectives in terms of the research questions, and clarify what the primary objective is. As we considered in Chapter 2, most clinical trials are interested in a difference in outcome between treatment groups. One major exception is an early phase drug trial, which aims to find the appropriate dose for a treatment and/or focuses solely on safety (see Chapter 1 for a discussion of the different types of trials). We will consider this type of trial briefly towards the end of this chapter.

For most of this chapter, we will focus on the most common type of clinical trials, those comparing treatment groups (e.g. RCTs and comparative non-randomized clinical trials). To aid readability we will also refer to a standard RCT design though it should be noted the same calculations are relevant for clinical trials which are non-randomized if they are also seeking to compare the outcome between two groups, and if the groups are of equal size. Calculating the sample size for different types of clinical trials can be fairly technical and mathematical, and should be handled by someone with suitable training and expertise (such as a statistician). For those interested in reading in more depth about sample size calculations in general and also about other clinical trial designs, there are a number of good books available (2,3).

Purpose of the sample size calculation

The primary objective of a clinical trial is usually addressed in the statistical analysis by looking to see whether there is a difference between the treatments in a primary outcome (see Chapter 2). Correspondingly, the sample size of the trial is based upon detecting a difference in this primary outcome. For example, for a trial evaluating a new hypertension drug, a natural choice of primary outcome would be blood pressure (systolic and/or diastolic). Focusing on the primary outcome forces us to commit to a primary outcome, defining what the study's main result will be, and therefore what should ultimately be reported. We will discuss the statistical analysis and reporting of clinical trials in Chapters 9 and 10.

Sample size calculations are used to provide reassurance that if the data are successfully collected and analysed as planned, the study will likely answer the main research question. Usually this question is framed as what is called a *superiority* question: is there a difference in outcome between the treatment groups? The default answer (*null hypothesis*) is that there is no difference in outcome between the treatment groups. The statistical analysis looks for evidence that suggests this null hypothesis is wrong. Trials with this kind of research question can be described as a *superiority trial*. In contrast, an *equivalence*, or *non-inferiority*, *trial* asks a different question: do these treatments have the same (for an equivalence trial), or at least no worse (a non-inferiority trial), an outcome? The sample size calculation varies according to the kind of trial question we plan to answer. The knee replacement question we saw in Chapter 2 was framed as a superiority question, which is the most common way to express the research question.

The sample size calculation for a superiority trial seeks to ensure the pre-specified probability (*statistical power*) of detecting a statistical difference in the primary outcome of a certain magnitude (the *target difference*) is sufficiently high. We do not know whether there is a difference between the treatments in advance—that is why the study is being carried out. If there is a difference, we want to detect it, and the target difference is the value we are particularly interested in detecting. There is a possibility that we will make an error and miss it. Alternatively, there might not be a real difference between the treatments—there is therefore a risk by conducting the analysis that we falsely detect a spurious numerical difference when there is not a real one. Unfortunately, it is not possible to exclude the possibility of making both of these two errors. The best that can be achieved is to restrict them to pre-specified levels within the sample size calculation. The two *errors* are controlled by the pre-specified statistical significance level (type I error rate) and the statistical power (1 minus the type II error rate). The most critical input in the sample size calculation is the magnitude of the difference we wish to detect (target difference). Like life more generally, the more subtle a difference that we want to detect (i.e. the smaller the target difference), the more carefully we need to consider whether it is there or not. In this context, that means more data and therefore a larger sample size. The target difference should be one that is important to at least one of the key stakeholder groups for the clinical trials (e.g. patients, health professionals, or regulatory bodies). Commonly it is a difference that patients would consider important to them, and would help them choose between treatments, or not to have treatment at all. For example, a patient might well opt for a drug if it could reduce systolic blood pressure by 10 mmHg, if in turn this is associated with a 34% reduction in the risk of stroke (4).

Conventional approach to sample size calculations

Although there are different statistical approaches for calculating sample size, most trials, to the frustration of some statisticians, follow a *conventional approach* (5). The conventional approach is sometimes referred to as *Neyman–Pearson* after the two statisticians whose work coalesced to produce the approach. This way of conducing the sample size calculation is sometimes referred to as *statistical hypothesis testing*, reflecting the fact that a formal statistical test related to a specified (or at least implicit) hypothesis is part of the approach. It is also sometimes called a *power calculation*, reflecting the calculation of the statistical power for a given sample size, target difference, and significance level. Some researchers start by thinking about how many participants they think they can recruit, and then work 'backwards' to see what statistical power might be achieved. This backwards approach is not recommended. Instead, thinking about what we wish to detect is a more productive way to start the process.

The conventional approach to sample size calculation is not without limitations. However, to date none of the alternatives have gained substantial use (see 'Other approaches to sample size determination' later in this chapter). Under the conventional approach, the required sample size is dependent on a number of factors:

1. The trial design.
2. The type of outcome to be analysed.
3. The intended statistical analysis.
4. The statistical parameters: statistical significance level and statistical power.
5. The target difference: the difference in outcome between the two treatment groups that we want to detect (expressed differently according to points 2 and 3).

We will focus on the standard trial design, which can be more formally described as a two-arm parallel group randomized trial with a 1:1 allocation ratio. We will now consider how to calculate the sample size for the three main outcome types in turn: continuous, binary, or time-to-event outcomes. Three worked examples (one for each of the main outcome types) are given in the subsequent sections of this chapter to illustrate how sample size calculations for clinical trials work in practice and to show the impact of varying different inputs. However, while these and other formulae can be used to calculate by hand the required number, checking the calculation against a validated program, and seeking advice from an expert, is highly recommended prior to confirming the sample size.

Continuous outcome

Sample size for a continuous outcome under a standard trial design

A commonly used formula (2) to estimate the number needed per group for a superiority trial with a continuous outcome (y) is:

$$n = \frac{2\left(Z_{1-\beta} + Z_{1-\alpha/2}\right)^2 \sigma^2}{\delta^2} + \frac{Z_{1-\alpha/2}^2}{4} \qquad (5.1)$$

where $Z_{1-\beta}$ and $Z_{1-\alpha/2}$ refer to the values from the standard normal distribution (i.e. a normal distribution with a mean of zero and standard deviation of one) for which the probability of exceeding it is $1-\beta$ and $1-\alpha/2$ respectively. $1-\beta$ is the statistical power and α is the statistical significance level. The division of α by 2 indicates we are planning a two-sided statistical test. σ is the population standard deviation, and δ is the target difference here defined as a difference in the means of intervention group ($\bar{y}_I$) and the control group ($\bar{y}_C$) observations, that is, $\bar{y}_I - \bar{y}_C$ Variants on this formula are in use. In practice, σ is typically assumed to be known, with an estimate from an existing study used as if it were the population value. Formulas which allow for statistical uncertainty regarding σ are available (2).

The use of formula 5.1 requires a number of assumptions:

1. There are two groups of individuals who will each receive one of the two treatments (I and C), that is, a standard (individually randomized parallel group) trial design.
2. We are interested in whether or not the treatments differ, that is, if the intervention is better than the control or if the control is better than the intervention is of interest to us. In other words, our interest is whether the intervention is superior to the control *or* whether the control is superior to the intervention treatment. We describe the resulting analysis as two-sided, and hence why we divided α by 2 in formula 5.1.
3. The treatment groups are of equal size (i.e. 1:1 randomization allocation ratio will be used).
4. The outcome is not only continuous, it is also normally distributed.
5. We know what level of variability in the outcome to expect.
6. The statistical analysis will be carried out using an independent t-test (or equivalent).

The sample size generated tells you the number of observations needed in the statistical analysis. This number is not necessarily the same as the number recruited to the clinical trial, as there may well be participants for whom data will not ultimately be available (see Chapter 9 for discussion of the practical consequences of this in the statistical analysis). We now turn to a worked example using formula 5.1.

Worked example—continuous outcome under a standard trial design

Let us assume we are interested in carrying out a randomized trial to evaluate a new antihypertensive drug that we will compare against a placebo control for patients with hypertension. The primary outcome is systolic blood pressure measured after 12 weeks on the drug (either the intervention or the control). From our experience, we consider a mean reduction of 10 mmHg to be clinically important as noted above, so have chosen this to be the *target difference*. Based on previous literature, we anticipate that the variability (*standard deviation*) in the systolic blood pressure measurement will be 20 mmHg. For 80% statistical power and two-sided 5% statistical significance level using formula 5.1 we have:

$$n = \frac{2\left(0.84 + 1.96^2\right)20^2}{10^2} + \frac{1.96^2}{4} = 64 \; per \; group$$

The values of 0.84 and 1.96 above are the standard normal distribution (Z) values for statistical power of 80% (i.e. Z value of 0.84) and a two-sided 5% significance level (i.e. Z value of 1.96). Based upon all of the inputs stated above, a sample size of 64 individuals per group (i.e. 128 overall) is required for the statistical analysis. We can see the impact of 12 different scenarios (with different combinations of input values) in Table 5.1; the example we have just calculated is scenario 5. The target difference, standard deviation, and statistical power are varied across the scenarios while the significance level is kept at the same level. If the standard deviation in the systolic blood pressure measurement was in fact 25 mm Hg, then the required sample size will increase to 99 per group (scenario 6). If we can reduce the variability in this measurement to 15 mmHg, perhaps with better equipment and training of the staff taking the measurements, then the sample size required will decrease to 36 per group (scenario 4). Similar changes could be made to each of the inputs. The standard normal Z value for 90% power is 1.28, which

Table 5.1 Systolic blood pressure continuous outcome example: sample size scenarios

Scenario	Target difference (mmHg)	Standard deviation (mmHg)	Statistical significance level	Statistical power	Required sample size (per group)
1	5	15	5% (2-sided)	80%	142
2	5	20	5% (2-sided)	80%	252
3	5	25	5% (2-sided)	80%	393
4	10	15	5% (2-sided)	80%	36
5	10	20	5% (2-sided)	80%	64
6	10	25	5% (2-sided)	80%	99
7	5	15	5% (2-sided)	90%	190
8	5	20	5% (2-sided)	90%	337
9	5	25	5% (2-sided)	90%	526
10	10	15	5% (2-sided)	90%	48
11	10	20	5% (2-sided)	90%	85
12	10	25	5% (2-sided)	90%	132

when include in formula 5.1 will always give a higher sample size for 90% power than for 80% power when the other inputs remain the same. The key point to draw from this set of scenarios is that what seem to be plausible and sensible changes in the inputs can dramatically alter the required sample size, from 36 per group to 526 per group. We can see the impact more generally on the sample size required of varying the target difference, standard deviation, statistical power, and significance level values while keeping all the other values constant (as per scenario 5) in Figure 5.1. Three key things can be clearly seen in the four graphs. First, the increase in the sample size is not even across the respective ranges (i.e. the relationships are curves and not straight lines). For example, the incremental increase in the sample size moving from a standard deviation of 15 to 20 is only 27 per group, whereas the increase moving from a standard deviation of 45 to 50 is 75 per group. Second, the impact of varying the different inputs is not the same. The shape of the four curves is clearly different. For two inputs (target difference and statistical significance level), the larger the value, the smaller the sample size needed, whereas for statistical power and variance, the larger the value, the larger the sample size needed. Third, different combinations of input values can lead to the same sample size. For example, all four curves have a point where the number required per group is 100. An implication of this is that we need to record all of the inputs when we conduct a sample size calculation, and report accordingly (5).

(a)
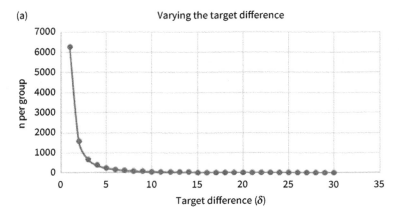

(b)
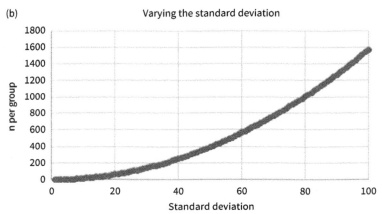

(c)
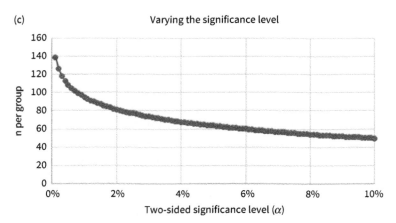

Figure 5.1 Impact on the sample size of varying different parameters for a continuous outcome—worked example (scenario 5).

(d)

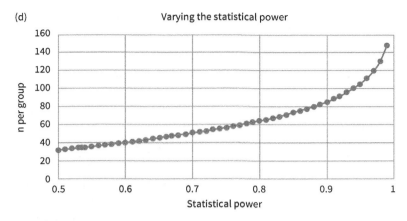

Figure 5.1 Continued

Binary outcome

Sample size for a binary outcome under a standard trial design

A binary outcome is one where there are only two possible responses (i.e. yes or no, event or no event). The approach to calculating the sample size is very similar to that of a continuous outcome. A different formula is used to reflect the difference in the outcome and intended analysis. Commonly, a formula that corresponds to an analysis using a (Pearson's) chi-squared test is used. For a standard RCT design (two arms, 1:1 randomization) addressing again a superiority question we have:

$$n = \frac{\left(z_{1-\frac{\alpha}{2}} + z_{1-\beta}\right)^2 \left(p_I\left(1-p_I\right) + p_C\left(1-p_C\right)\right)}{\left(p_I - p_C\right)^2} \tag{5.2}$$

where n is the required number of observations in each of the two randomized groups, and $Z_{1-\beta}$ and $Z_{1-\alpha/2}$ refer to values from the standard (i.e. one with a mean of 0 and standard deviation of 1) normal distribution as before. p_I and p_C are the anticipated probability of an event in intervention and control treatment groups, respectively. α is the statistical significance level (i.e. the type I error rate), and β is the type II error rate and is chosen so that $1 - \beta$ is equal to the desired statistical power. Formula 5.2 makes the same implicit assumptions numbered 1–3 as given above for the continuous outcome. Here of course we assume a binary outcome, and that we can state the target difference as the difference in the probability of an event in two groups. We also assume an appropriate analysis will be carried out (e.g. Pearson chi-squared test as the above calculation directly relates to, and perhaps also using a 95% confidence interval for the difference in proportions). As for the continuous outcome formula 5.1, the number produced by formula 5.2 is the number of observations analysed. Therefore, we will have to increase the sample size if we expect any missing data.

The similarity in formula 5.2 to formula 5.1 is not accidental. The difference in the proportions between the groups $p_I - p_C$ defines the target difference as an absolute difference in proportions, for example, if p_I and p_C were 0.2 and 0.3 respectively, it would be −0.1. The response from a binary outcome (i.e. binomial distribution) in each group is converted so that it approximates one from a normal distribution assuming the sample size is sufficiently 'large'. The corresponding test to analyse the data uses this approximation to derive a test for how unlikely the observed data are (using the chi-squared distribution, hence the name 'chi-squared test'). We again consider an example to illustrate how we can calculate the sample size for a binary outcome.

Worked example—binary outcome under a standard trial design

A randomized trial to evaluate the use of adalimumab in addition to routine care over a control group of routine care only for elderly individuals in a care home with severe acute respiratory syndrome coronavirus 2 (SARS-CoV-2) was planned early in the COVID-19 pandemic. The main outcome of interest was the occurrence of serious or critical illness, or death within 28 days. Based upon a previous study of 72,431 individuals with the disease in China (6), an event risk of 0.19 (i.e. 19 out of 100 individuals would experience the event) was considered realistic for the control (usual care) group. At the time, a target difference of a reduction in the proportion of events to 0.09 (i.e. 9 out of 100 individuals) was felt appropriate. Given the potential side effects of the drug, a substantial effect would be needed to warrant use in practice. As before, we can look at the impact upon the potential sample size of varying the assumptions in the calculation, the statistical power, and the proportions in each group.

Table 5.2 provides the required number per group using formula 5.2 for 12 credible scenarios for this trial. This bases the routine care group event proportion upon the data from the Chinese study and the target difference of 0.1

Table 5.2 COVID-19 binary outcome example: sample size scenarios

Scenario	Target difference (absolute difference)	Routine care group	Adalimumab group	Statistical significance level	Statistical power	Required sample size (per group)
1	0.10	0.19	0.09	5% (2-sided)	80%	185
2	0.07	0.19	0.12	5% (2-sided)	80%	416
3	0.10	0.25	0.15	5% (2-sided)	80%	247
4	0.07	0.25	0.18	5% (2-sided)	80%	537
5	0.10	0.15	0.05	5% (2-sided)	80%	137
6	0.07	0.15	0.08	5% (2-sided)	80%	322
7	0.10	0.19	0.09	5% (2-sided)	90%	248
8	0.07	0.19	0.12	5% (2-sided)	90%	556
9	0.10	0.25	0.15	5% (2-sided)	90%	331
10	0.07	0.25	0.18	5% (2-sided)	90%	719
11	0.10	0.15	0.05	5% (2-sided)	90%	184
12	0.07	0.15	0.08	5% (2-sided)	90%	431

reduction (therefore a proportion of 0.09 in the intervention group), with two-sided statistical significance level and statistical power of 80% (scenario 1 in Table 5.2) requires 185 per group ($185 \times 2 = 370$ overall). This can be calculated by hand using formula 5.2 as:

$$n = \frac{(0.84 + 1.96)^2 \left(0.19(1 - 0.19) + 0.09(1 - 0.09)\right)}{(0.09 - 0.19)^2} = 185 \text{ per group}$$

As for a continuous outcome, as the target difference is reduced, the sample size required increases. In scenario 2, the target difference is reduced to 0.07 by increasing the adalimumab group level while keeping the other inputs the same. This leads to a dramatic increase to 416 per group (more than double) for a relatively minor adjustment in the target difference (scenario 2). Using statistical power of 90% for target differences of 0.10 and 0.07 reduction but keeping the routine care level at 0.19 as before, gives the higher numbers of 248 and 556 (scenarios 7 and 8) as anticipated.

Less intuitive is that the sample size required for a binary outcome differs according to the relative proportion levels as well as absolute target difference. Smaller sample sizes are required the further away the proportions are from 0.5. Corresponding number per group required with a higher event proportion of 0.25 instead of 0.19 for the routine group (but the same target differences of 0.10 and 0.07) requires 331 and 719 per group for 90% statistical power (scenarios 9 and 10). If the event proportion in the routine care group is, however, lower at say 0.15, then only 184 and 431 per group are required for corresponding target differences (scenarios 11 and 12). Corresponding numbers for 80% statistical power can also be calculated (scenarios 1–6). The range of potential samples in this summary illustrates the great sensitivity to minor variations in the inputs. For the 12 scenarios considered here, the required number per group ranged from 137 to 719 (i.e. the highest sample size was over five times larger than the smallest).

Target differences for binary outcomes

In the previous example we used an absolute difference between the proportions in each group to express the target difference (i.e. the difference we wished to be confident we would be able to detect). An absolute difference directly links to formula 5.2. The impact of varying the target difference can be readily seen as the smaller the difference gets, the larger the overall sample size will get. For example, halving this absolute target difference using formula 5.2 will lead to a quadrupling of the required sample size as the denominator in the formula will reduce to a quarter. Nevertheless, to fully (i.e. uniquely) express the target difference for a binary outcome sample size calculation, the control (reference) group level needs to be given, that is, an absolute reduction in the proportion of critical, serious illness, or morality of *0.1 from 0.19* (i.e. from 0.19 to 0.09).

The quantification of the treatment effect of a binary outcome is often expressed in two other ways rather than as a risk difference. It can also be expressed as a risk ratio (RR) or as an odds ratio (OR). The former is simply the ratio of the risk or proportion of anticipated events (i.e. P_I / P_C). The odds ratio is the ratio of the odds in the intervention group to the control group, and

can be calculated as $\dfrac{(P_I / (1-(P_I)))}{(P_C / (1-P_C))}$. An OR or RR might link more naturally

than the risk difference to the intended statistical analysis. Whichever one is used, as when expressing the target difference as a risk difference, the control group level needs to be given to fully specify the target difference. It is worth noting that different sample size formulas can be used instead of the one we have considered above including some which directly relate to analyses that produce different treatment effect size measures (e.g. OR instead of the risk difference). It is useful to note that for the most likely range of OR values to be considered in an RCT (ORs 0.3–3.0), the relationship of the absolute risk difference (ignoring the sign, i.e. whether it is positive or negative) to the value of the OR is:

$$Absolute\,(P_I - P_C) = Absolute\,(log_e\,(OR))\,p_{average}\,(1 - p_{average})$$

where $p_{average} = \dfrac{P_I + P_C}{2}$, that is, the average of the event proportions in the intervention and control groups (2). The OR and the RR will only be similar when the event proportions are very low (e.g. 0.05 or less). As such low proportions of events tend to lead to very large sample sizes and therefore are unlikely to be a practical option for a clinical trial, sample size calculations for RRs and ORs in practice cannot be considered interchangeable.

Time-to-event outcome

Sample size for a time-to-event outcome under a standard design

Time-to-event outcomes are like binary outcomes in that they use data on the occurrence of an event (that either occurred or it did not) for participants. However, they differ in that they also define the time for which the outcome has been assessed. The final status is thus either the occurrence of an event or is 'censored' by a particular time point. The length of this follow-up is allowed to vary between participants unlike for a binary variable where we assume a consistent time point. Time-to-event outcomes are often referred to as 'survival' outcomes given their original use for assessing mortality. For each participant, they either died during the follow-up or they 'survived' up to a specific time point. This general approach is now used for a range of different events, hence the term time-to-event outcomes. For example, a very common one in cardiology studies is called MACE (major adverse cardiac events) (7). When this outcome is analysed as a time-to-event outcome, the analysis assesses the first occurrence of any one of a variety of cardiovascular-related episodes (irrespective of whether it is a stroke or myocardial infarction, for example,), as an event, as well as mortality.

The sample size calculation approach is roughly similar to a binary outcome though the intended use of a time-to-event analysis leads to multiple ways (and implied degrees of knowledge) of expressing the pattern of events in both treatment groups over the follow-up time. For simplicity, one of the most common approaches is to calculate the sample size based upon conducting a comparison of the survival curves (i.e. plotting the occurrence of events over time for each group and looking for statistical evidence of a difference between these curves). The typical statistical test used is called a log-rank test. A corresponding sample size can be calculated by defining the curves by giving the expected proportion of events in each group at the same point in time. For example, we may expect 0.2 of individuals in the intervention treatment group to experience an event and 0.3 of individuals to experience an event in the control group after 5 years of follow-up. An additional assumption is commonly made called 'proportional hazards'. It can be thought of as assuming a constant effect of the intervention treatment relative to the control treatment (or vice versa) over the period that participants are in the study. This implies that the 'hazard' of an event in the intervention treatment group relative to the control group is constant over time. In other words, there is not a situation where one treatment works better than the other early on but not so later on (or vice versa). By making this assumption of a constant treatment effect, the number of events that are needed to be observed for the required level of statistical power and significance level can be calculated more straightforwardly. The treatment effect can be also be expressed as the hazard ratio (HR) of one treatment to another. The HR can be calculated given the probability in each group as the ratio of the logarithms of the survival probabilities (S_I and S_C) in the respective group:

$$HR = \frac{ln(S_I)}{ln(S_C)} \tag{5.3}$$

A commonly used formula to calculate the overall number of events (E) is (8):

$$E = \left(z_{1-\frac{\alpha}{2}} + z_{1-\beta} \right)^2 \left(\frac{HR+1}{HR-1} \right)^2 \tag{5.4}$$

where $Z_{1-\beta}$ and $Z_{1-\alpha/2}$ refer to values from the standard (i.e. one with a mean of 0 and standard deviation of 1) normal distribution, $1-\beta$ is the statistical power and α is the statistical significance level, and HR and can be calculated using formula 5.3.

From this we can get the number of participants we need to recruit to our trial. In the case of the same follow-up period for all participants we have:

$$N \ per \ group = \frac{E}{(2 - S_I - S_C)} \tag{5.5}$$

As with formula 5.1 used for a continuous outcome, we have made a number of assumptions by using formula 5.5:

> We have implicitly made the same first three assumptions (1–3) as previously stated for a continuous outcome as well as three more:
> 1. A standard trial design.
> 2. Two-sided comparison.
> 3. Equal group sizes.
> 4. We have assumed there can only be one event (e.g. death) or at least we are only interested in the first one that occurs. For death that is clearly fine but for other events this is less satisfactory. For example, the commonly used composite outcome MACE includes a stroke as an event as well as cardiovascular death but we will also be interested if those who have a stroke later died due to cardiovascular disease within the follow-up period.
> 5. Constant HR
> 6. The formula addresses missing data due to (random) censoring. Missing data due to other reasons other than not observing the event in the follow-up period, for example, participant withdrawal, would need to be compensated for by increasing the sample size.

Various refinements of the sample size calculation given in formulas 5.3–5.5 can be made. These include making specific assumptions about the distribution of events (expected pattern of events over the follow-up period) in each group, and allowing for varying lengths of follow-up between participants due to censoring and the impact of the period of recruitment. Details on corresponding calculations are provided elsewhere (2).

Worked example—time-to-event outcome under a standard trial design

The Arterial Revascularisation Trial (ART) (9) was a randomized trial of bilateral versus single internal mammary artery graft surgery for coronary heart disease. It is a common operation, and it was estimated at the time there were 800,000 operations worldwide per year. Coronary artery bypass graft surgery was conventionally carried out using a single arterial graft along with supplemental grafts. However, the grafted arteries can become blocked over time and the patient may require further treatment over subsequent years including repeat surgery. The use of two (bilateral) arteries to improve patient survival and avoid further treatment (including a repeat coronary artery bypass graft) had been proposed. Nine previous studies had been carried out, of varying sizes and degrees of methodological rigour, to compare the two surgical approaches (bilateral versus single internal mammary graft) though none had used an RCT design. Together, they suggested the possibility of a substantial reduction in mortality with the bilateral graft operation. Table 5.3 shows 12 scenarios for the sample size calculation for this trial (9). The HR, the number of events, and the number of patients required are calculated using formulas 5.3–5.5 for various possible levels of survival in the single and bilateral groups. If we again have two-sided statistical significance of 5% and statistical power of 80%, and use survival proportions of 0.85 and 0.75, we require 102 events which leads to 254 individuals per group (scenario 1).

It is interesting to note that different combinations of two survival proportions can lead to the same target HR. For example, a HR of 0.73 is produced by scenarios 2 and 4. Similarly, different combinations can produce the same absolute target difference (e.g. 0.05 for scenarios 5 and 6), but never both. As before, the smaller the target difference (e.g. a HR closer to 1.0 or an absolute difference closer to 0), the larger the sample size that is needed. Halving the absolute target difference to 0.05 from 0.1 (bilateral remaining at 0.85, i.e. scenario 2 instead of 1), leads to more than three times as many events being required (908 instead of 254). As before, like for like (e.g. scenario 1 versus 7, etc.), as the statistical power is increased from 80% to 90%, the required number of events and ultimately the sample size required have increased. The final sample size selected for the study was 3000 individuals and followed scenario 11 (rounding up a little for the final figure). That is an absolute target difference of a 5% (or 0.05 in proportions) reduction in the mortality at 10 years between the two groups with respective survival proportions of 0.85 and 0.80, two-sided statistical significance, and statistical power at 90%.

Which input values to use?

As we have seen, minor changes in the inputs can lead to very different sample sizes. Therefore, the input values we use matter greatly. Each of the main inputs is considered in turn.

For a statistically significant level, the use of a two-sided 5% level is ubiquitous despite it being an arbitrary choice. However, it has probably lasted as it is not a terrible choice. Furthermore, if it were to change it would typically be

Table 5.3 Arterial Revascularisation Trial time-to-event outcome example: sample size scenarios

Scenario	Single approach survival at 10 years	Bilateral approach survival at 10 years	Absolute difference	Hazard ratio	Statistical significance level	Statistical power	Number of events	Sample size (per group)
1	0.75	0.85	0.1	0.56	5% (2-sided)	80%	102	254
2	0.8	0.85	0.05	0.73	5% (2-sided)	80%	318	908
3	0.75	0.82	0.07	0.69	5% (2-sided)	80%	233	542
4	0.75	0.81	0.06	0.73	5% (2-sided)	80%	329	748
5	0.75	0.8	0.05	0.78	5% (2-sided)	80%	492	1093
6	0.7	0.75	0.05	0.81	5% (2-sided)	80%	685	1245
7	0.75	0.85	0.1	0.56	5% (2-sided)	90%	136	340
8	0.8	0.85	0.05	0.73	5% (2-sided)	90%	425	1215
9	0.75	0.82	0.07	0.69	5% (2-sided)	90%	312	725
10	0.75	0.81	0.06	0.73	5% (2-sided)	90%	441	1002
11	0.75	0.8	0.05	0.78	5% (2-sided)	90%	658	1463
12	0.7	0.75	0.05	0.81	5% (2-sided)	90%	917	1666

to a lower value, given what we know about the potential for false findings (see Chapter 9). This though would result in larger sample sizes, and given many clinical trials fail to meet their intended recruited sample size, there is little appetite for such a change. In trials with alternative trial designs, or with more complex analyses, individual comparisons may have differing levels for statistical significance in order to maintain an overall 5% significance. Decisions about when and how this should be done are open to critique and debate (10).

Values used for statistical power are rarely anything other than 80% or 90%. While even higher would be desirable as the statistical power approaches 100%, the growth in the sample size per percentage increase in power goes up rapidly (as can be seen in Figure 5.1). As a consequence, except for the largest of target differences (or the most precisely measured outcomes), statistical power beyond 95% tends to results in very large, typically prohibitively large, sample sizes. The marginal gain is relatively small.

This brings us to the outcome-specific inputs. These are the mean difference and standard deviation for a continuous outcome. For a binary outcome they are the intervention and control group risks at a specific point in time. The survival probability in both groups, with or without a HR, are the corresponding inputs for a time-to-event outcome. These fix the target difference in the corresponding outcome. There are rightly no universal conventions. Why this is the case is easy to see. For example, for our COVID-19 binary example, 0.19 of the routine care group were anticipated to have a serious or critical illness, and/ or die within 28 days. Suppose we decided to conduct the study in a primary (family doctor) care setting instead of a care home setting. The age of the likely participants would in general be much younger (median of about 39 years in England and Wales) (11) than in care homes where 83% of the population (2011 figures) (12) are 65 years or over. The event rate that would be realistic for this younger, and likely healthier population would be much lower. How much so is difficult to predict but morality alone appeared at the time to vary greatly by age group with less than 1% in under 20-year-olds to over 10% for those aged 80 years plus at the point of considering this trial. Furthermore, the target difference of 0.1 which was considered appropriate for the care home setting may also no longer be credible. A realistic absolute difference value for this population would be somewhat lower, perhaps so much so that the trial is no longer considered feasible in that setting. Additionally, these values all look (thankfully) very high now given the substantial improvements made in treatment patients with COVID-19. So if we were to conduct this study now, the expected survival rates would be much higher even for older, and sicker participants.

Hopefully what is clear from the above example is that the sample size cannot be considered in isolation from other key aspects of the study design, including the PICOTS along with recruitment, data collection, and follow-up.

Furthermore, it fits a specific time period particularly for a binary time-to-event outcome over time. As noted in Chapter 2, the trial design might be best thought of as like sculpting, where the overall vision needs to be kept in mind to avoid going awry, as one is tempted to chip away here and there. When it comes to determining the sample size, as Bradford Hill noted in 1952, there can be no magic number either for the statistician or for health professionals, or, one might add, for patients (1). We have to reflect on the impact of choices regarding the sample size on the trial design as a whole.

Allowing for missing data

The formulas presented above do not make any allowance for missing data. For binary and continuous outcomes, to allow for missing data, the number needed for the analysis can be divided by the expected proportion of available data. For example, if 142 per group were needed as per scenario 1 in Table 5.1 and 10% of the data was expected to be missing the number to recruit would be $142/.9 = 158$ per group. Similarly for scenario 3 in Table 5.2 but allowing for 20% missing data we need $247/.8 = 309$ per group. For a time to event outcome the same approach could be used though typically we would make a more nuanced allowance for loss of data over the time period of interest. Details are provided elsewhere (2).

Other approaches to sample size determination

Overview

The previous sections have all presumed a standard trial design, that is, an RCT with two evenly sized groups seeking to address a superiority question. Use of an alternative trial design, including as simple a change as using a different randomization allocation ratio other than 1:1, will require adjustment to the calculations presented earlier. Similarly, use of a trial design such as a cluster or a crossover trial design will also require different calculations. The process can sometimes be carried out in a similar manner and with the same underlying statistical approach followed by making an adjustment. In Chapter 4 we considered simple adjustments to deal with some alternative trial designs. These can be applied to the value from the relevant formulas provided in this chapter to address the different trial design.

The conventional approach to sample size calculations has been criticized as both too simplistic, and also confusing to non-statisticians. Furthermore, reviews of practice have consistently highlighted errors in calculations, and misunderstanding (13). There are a number of different statistical approaches which could instead be adopted when determining the sample size for a clinical trial. In-depth discussion of these is beyond the scope of this book but interested readers can look for an introduction to these topics and a primer to the sizable corresponding literature elsewhere (5,14,15). In this section the most common alternative statistical approaches are briefly presented.

Sample size determination for clinical trials focused upon safety

Early phase (1 and 2) drug clinical trials may not seek to provide even a provisional assessment of the treatment effect. Instead, they may be focused on safety and in particular quantifying toxicity. The specific focus of such a study may be to identify the MTD. Accordingly, the design including the sample size of the study should reflect this primary objective. The study sample size may not in fact be a fixed figure as is the case under a conventional sample size as described earlier in this chapter. Instead, there may be a maximum number of participants for the study—the actual number recruited being dependent upon the recruited patients' data and specifically the occurrence of adverse safety events. Consideration then is focused upon defining the process by which the dose level is varied in order to identify the MTD, and confirming the maximum number of participants. Accordingly, the study may stop early if the MTD is identified early or continuation will not lead to the MTD being identified. For early phase trials of drugs, the events of interest are often referred to as toxicity-limiting events—those which will lead us to restricting the dose used in the study and ultimately the recommended dose for use in any subsequent clinical trial. Corresponding trial designs typically follow one of two approaches: i) those with pre-set options in terms of the possible dose levels and the potential number of individuals receiving them (rule-based approach); and ii) those which are based upon statistical modelling of the dose level and corresponding probability of a toxicity event given the accumulating data (model-based approaches) (16).

Probably the most common dose escalation design belonging to the rule-based approach is the '3 + 3' design. Under this design three individuals are given the initial dose. Three more individuals may be given the same dose if one of the initial three experiences a toxicity event; a higher dose will be given to the next three if none of the three experience a toxicity event. Alternatively, the study may stop if more than one individual experiences a toxicity-related adverse event. The maximum number of individuals at each dose level is usually two sets of three (i.e. six individuals). If only one or none experience a toxicity event at this dose level then the process repeats for the next pre-specified higher dose. Otherwise the study stops and the MTD may or may not be declared to be identified depending upon the number of toxicity events identified in the final dose. The range of possible sample sizes is then a function of the number of different dose levels that have been pre-specified for the study. As a consequence, the choice of dose levels, in particular the initial levels, are of critical importance. For example, for the standard 3 + 3 design, the minimum number of participants in the study is only three while the maximum number receiving each dose level is six. The maximum number of individuals overall is six times the number of doses which could be used in the study (e.g. a 3 + 3 design with four dose levels can have up to 4 × 6 = 24 participants). While simple to understand and to implement, the 3 + 3 design has been criticized for its potential to fail to correctly identify the MTD (both substantially under-estimating the MTD and overestimating it). This risk is altered by the quality of the pre-specified dose levels, especially the initial levels, which are to be used. Accordingly, various adaptations of this design have been proposed including a change in the number who receive the drug dose at the same level.

More satisfying, to a pharmacologist and a statistician at least, is to design the study to estimate the underlying relationship between the dose an individual receives and the probability of them experiencing a toxicity-related adverse event. By doing this we can respond to the data as they become available (after each participant's data). This will hopefully increase the chance of selecting the correct dose as the MTD prior to the study's conclusion. This second type of design (model-based approach) uses an underlying assumed model to determine the dose level to choose for the next individual. Figure 5.2 shows an example based upon assuming a particular type of curve relationship (logistic)

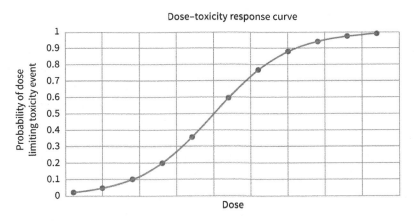

Figure 5.2 Dose–toxicity response curve—modelling approach.

between the possible doses (shown as squares) and the probability of an individual experiencing a toxicity event. Happily, in this example, the initial dose (first square) has a probability of only 0.02 (2 in 100). This probability increases as we progress through the dose levels (the fourth dose has a probability of 0.20 (1 in 5); the highest dose (final square) has one of 0.99 (99 in 100). The continual reassessment method, proposed in the 1990s, sought to assess the most appropriate dose for each subsequent patient after the initial one, in order to find the MTD (defined as the probability of a severe toxicity adverse event being no higher than the desired level, say 0.2). Various mathematical forms can be used to model the dose–toxicity relationships (14) but the sample size is then typically capped at a level which is viewed as organizationally manageable, and financially acceptable. It should also be one which will provide good statistical operating characteristics (i.e. a high probability of finding the optimal dose level, minimizing the number experiencing toxicity events and the likely sample size, etc.). Determining this maximum sample size, and confirming the appropriateness of the assumed model, typically involves carrying out a simulation study (i.e. carrying out a run of a large number of hypothetical trials, perhaps 10,000, for which a plausible dose–toxicity response curve is assumed). What happens at the end of each simulated study is observed so that the overall pattern of statistical characteristics can be estimated. An overview of the findings from these hypothetical trials provides insight into what could occur, and what is likely to happen, should the simulated scenario play out. It is also worth noting that simultaneous assessment of safety and efficacy is possible and the sample size could be determined accordingly though this adds further complexity (17,18). Further consideration is beyond the scope of this book.

Precision-based approach

A distinctly different approach to sample size calculation from what we have considered so far is a precision-based one. The RCT sample size calculations have been premised on controlling the type I and II errors by using pre-set values for the statistical significance and power. The early phase calculation discussed above focused on safety events and identifying the optimal dose. Alternatively, the statistical aim of the study could be expressed as achieving a desired level of precision when estimating the object of interest (e.g. the mean difference in systolic blood pressure between treatments). Provided we also specify a degree of statistical certainty as well (significance level), we can readily calculate the number of individuals needed in each group. This statistical precision can be expressed in a confidence interval, typically 95%, and quantified by the width of the interval. For example a 95% confidence interval for the difference in systolic blood pressure which ranges from −40 to 20 mmHg (i.e. a width of 60 mmHg) might be considered of little clinical use. However, one which has a width of only 10 mmHg (e.g. 5–15 mmHg) may well be considered useful. The number of individuals needed in each group to achieve this can be calculated in a similar manner to before, if we have an understanding of the expected level of variation in the measurement of systolic blood pressure in mmHg that we expect. Similar considerations as for choosing the target difference of interest can help fix the desired width. Simple calculations for common situations are provided elsewhere (19).

This precision approach can be adopted for other types of clinical trials, for example, if a preliminary assessment of efficacy response is desired in a single group (i.e. there is no control) phase 1 trial. The same precision-focused approach could be adopted but this time for the absolute level of the treatment group's response. Some phase 1 trials include a small cohort of patients who receive the recommended dose based upon the phase 1 dose-escalation study. In this context, a sufficient number of patients could be recruited to the 'extension cohort' to give reassurance that drug activity is in keeping with the desired level. For example, if the proportion of patients responding is thought to be 0.70, only 24 individuals are required to have a 90% confidence interval (Wilson's method) that would exclude proportions lower than 0.55. A formula to show this is given elsewhere (20). Another type of clinical trial for which a precision-based approach is popular is for pilot or feasibility trials where the key outcomes of interest are not the treatment effects in clinical outcomes but the measures characterizing key aspects of the study's conduct, such as the proportion of individuals receiving the randomly allocated treatment (i.e. compliance). This calculation can be conducted in a similar manner.

Bayesian statistics

Bayesian statistical approaches to the sample size provide another quite different approach to those discussed so far. The general approach owes its name to the Reverend Thomas Bayes, who lived in 18th-century England and whose paper on what is called Bayes theorem was published after his death. Bayes theorem is given in formula 5.6:

$$Pr(A \mid B) = \frac{Pr(B \mid A)Pr(A)}{Pr(B)} \tag{5.5}$$

In this formula A and B represent two different events, with $Pr(A), Pr(B), Pr(A \mid B), and\ Pr(B \mid A)$ presenting the probabilities of A, B, A given B, and B given A, respectively. Bayes theorem states how to update an existing estimate of the probability of an event $((\Pr(A)$ as presented in formula 5.6) based upon new data. Its application to simple probabilities of event for which reliable (prior) estimates of $\Pr(B)$ and $\Pr(A)$ are available such as for the performance of diagnostic tests is uncontroversial. Applying this approach more broadly has led to a quite different, arguably more intuitive, way to formulating statistical analyses. While the estimates of these prior probabilities could be based upon existing data (e.g. from a previous research study), they can be based upon belief alone or some synthesis of belief and prior data. This shift, though, has not been without controversy, moving the analysis in a more subjective direction. In the fuller form, we begin with an existing distribution for each variable of interest in the analysis (a prior distribution). The new data are then mathematically quantified (as a distribution) and used to update the previous view and provides a new estimate of the (now called the posterior) distribution relating to the quantity of interest (e.g. the difference in outcome between treatments). As might already be suspected, this can lead to complex mathematics in all but select, fairly simple scenarios. However, with the massive change in computing power over the last 30 years, many Bayesian computations are within the reach of a standard computer. Overall, the Bayesian framework is more flexible than the conventional statistical approach. In particular, it offers the potential to harness large data more efficiently. Use of Bayesian statistics is growing but it is still not that common in clinical research studies.

The use of Bayesian statistics in clinical trial sample size calculations has to date been concentrated in a number of key areas.

1. This approach has been used in clinical trial sample size determination for early phase trials which seek to identify the MTD (14). The continual reassessment method mentioned earlier was originally proposed in a Bayesian framework. The benefit of using a Bayesian approach is being able to directly utilize relevant prior evidence to inform the choice of the dose level for subsequent individuals and to identify the MTD in a model-based approach.

2. A Bayesian approach to sample size calculations has been used for phase 3 trial designs which will be analysed in the conventional way. The performance of a design and corresponding sample size can be considered against the conventional statistical parameters (i.e. controlling the type I and type II errors through the statistical significance level and statistical power). In this set-up, the Bayesian approach enables uncertainty related to key inputs (such as the variance of the systolic blood pressure measurement) to be readily incorporated into the calculation. To do so, a prior

distribution for the treatment difference has to be defined. A prior distribution for the treatment effect could be based upon previous studies (e.g. using pre-clinical data of a drug for the sample size calculation for a phase 3 trial of the same drug), and/or using expert opinion (21–23).

3. Fully Bayesian approaches to the sample size calculation of a phase 3 trial can also be carried out where the data are used as before but the assessment of the sufficiency of the sample size is based upon ensuring that there is a high predictive probability of meeting a pre-specified criterion for treatment success and/or failure. Alternatively, the focus can be upon the expected uncertainty associated with treatment effect and the corresponding credible interval (the Bayesian equivalent of a confidence interval). This latter approach is akin to the precision-based approach we discussed above but in a Bayesian framework.

4. Another area where Bayesian statistics are more commonly used in sample size determination for clinical trials is for adaptive trials (15). Assessments about adapting the design part way through the conduction of the study using the data accrued up to that point can be handled well using the flexibility of the approach, the ease with which predictive probabilities can be produced, and the natural fit with a decision-making approach. Similarly, alternating the allocation of treatments based upon acquired evidence is attractive in a Bayesian framework, utilizing the flexibility of the approach. The only 'cost' of Bayesian approach is the greater computation time, though this is less of an issue as processing power evolves. Underlying this though is the need to state upfront the prior distributions (i.e. quantify what is known at the outset to order to be able to formally quantify it after the new data are incorporated). If the prior distributions are poorly specified, it can undermine the benefit of the Bayesian approach.

Choosing the sample size

Choosing the sample size is one of the most critical decisions to make when designing a clinical trial. It impacts all aspects of the study. Given this, it is vital to carefully consider the implications of adopting a particular size of study. The appropriateness of a choice for the intended statistical analysis, and likelihood of producing findings that will influence key stakeholders (e.g. patients, healthcare professional, and regulators), should be considered, including in terms of the management and delivery of the study. The sample size should be sufficient to address the primary aim of the study (i.e. typically the analysis of the primary outcome). However, secondary concerns may also be of key importance. Possibilities include statistical analyses of other secondary outcomes, and planned analyses of a subset of participants focusing upon different outcomes or aspects. The collection of ancillary data may also influence the final choice to some degree. Consideration of a number of potential sample size options is prudent against the primary objective, and any key secondary objectives. Ultimately, there is no single 'right' sample size to be determined but there are many wrong (typically too small) sample sizes which will inhibit the objectives of the study being achieved. The main aim of a 'sample size calculation' therefore is to choose a sample size that is appropriate for the objective of the study while cognisant of the practical challenges that the sample size and intended trial design (including recruitment and data collection) will bring.

Summary

Determining the sample size is a critical aspect of a study, affecting the design, conduct, and analysis. Typically for an RCT this is done via a sample size calculation that focuses on a primary outcome which reflects the primary objective of the study. Under the conventional approach, a sample size should be large enough to ensure the desired target difference in the primary outcome is likely to be detected. The specific calculation varies according to the study design, primary outcome type, planned statistical analysis method, target difference in the primary outcome, and statistical parameters. Alternative approaches to the sample size determination are available which are suited to answering different questions (e.g. model-based approaches to estimating the MTD in an early phase drug clinical trial).

References

1. Hill AB. The clinical trial. New England Journal of Medicine. 1952;247:113–19.
2. Julious S. Sample Sizes for Clinical Trials. Boca Raton, FL: Chapman and Hall/CRC Press; 2010.
3. Daimon T, Hirakawa A, Matsui S. Dose-Finding Designs for Early-Phase Cancer Clinical Trials: A Brief Guidebook to Theory and Practice. Tokyo, Japan: Springer; 2019.
4. Law MR, Morris JK, Wald NJ. Use of blood pressure lowering drugs in the prevention of cardiovascular disease: meta-analysis of 147 randomised trials in the context of expectations from prospective epidemiological studies. BMJ. 2009;338:b1665.
5. Cook JA, Julious SA, Sones W, Hampson LV, Hewitt C, Berlin JA, et al. DELTA(2) guidance on choosing the target difference and undertaking and reporting the sample size calculation for a randomised controlled trial. BMJ. 2018;363:k3750.

6. Wu Z, McGoogan JM. Characteristics of and important lessons from the coronavirus disease 2019 (COVID-19) outbreak in China: summary of a report of 72 314 cases from the Chinese Center for Disease Control and Prevention. JAMA. 2020;323(13):1239–42.
7. Hupfeld C, Mudaliar S. Navigating the 'MACE' in cardiovascular outcomes trials and decoding the relevance of atherosclerotic cardiovascular disease benefits versus heart failure benefits. Diabetes, Obesity & Metabolism. 2019;21(8):1780–9.
8. Freedman LS. Tables of the number of patients required in clinical trials using the logrank test. Statistics in Medicine. 1982;1(2):121–9.
9. Taggart DP, Lees B, Gray A, Altman DG, Flather M, Channon K, et al. Protocol for the Arterial Revascularisation Trial (ART). A randomised trial to compare survival following bilateral versus single internal mammary grafting in coronary revascularisation [ISRCTN46552265]. Trials. 2006;7(1):7.
10. Wason JM, Stecher L, Mander AP. Correcting for multiple-testing in multi-arm trials: is it necessary and is it done? Trials. 2014;15:364.
11. Office for National Statistics. Age groups. 2020. Available from: https://www.ethnicity-facts-figures.service.gov.uk/uk-population-by-ethnicity/demographics/age-groups/latest
12. Office for National Statistics. Changes in the older resident care home population between 2001 and 2011. 2014. Available from: https://www.ons.gov.uk/peoplepopulationandcommunity/birthsdeathsandmarriages/ageing/articles/changesintheolderresidentcarehomepopulationbetween2001and2011/2014-08-01.
13. Copsey B, Thompson JY, Vadher K, Ali U, Dutton SJ, Fitzpatrick R, et al. Sample size calculations are poorly conducted and reported in many randomized trials of hip and knee osteoarthritis: results of a systematic review. Journal of Clinical Epidemiology. 2018;104:52–61.
14. Eisenhauer EA, Twelves C, Buyse M. Phase I Cancer Clinical Trials: A Practical Guide. 2nd ed. New York: Oxford University Press; 2015.
15. Berry SM. Bayesian Adaptive Methods for Clinical Trials. Boca Raton, FL: Chapman & Hall/CRC; 2010.
16. Wheeler GM, Mander AP, Bedding A, Brock K, Cornelius V, Grieve AP, et al. How to design a dose-finding study using the continual reassessment method. BMC Medical Research Methodology. 2019;19(1):18.
17. Mandrekar SJ, Qin R, Sargent DJ. Model-based phase I designs incorporating toxicity and efficacy for single and dual agent drug combinations: methods and challenges. Statistics in Medicine. 2010;29(10):1077–83.
18. Lin R, Yin G. STEIN: a simple toxicity and efficacy interval design for seamless phase I/II clinical trials. Statistics in Medicine. 2017;36(26):4106–20.
19. Cook JA, Julious SA, Sones W, Hampson LV, Hewitt C, Berlin JA, et al. Practical help for specifying the target difference in sample size calculations for RCTs: the DELTA(2) five-stage study, including a workshop. Health Technology Assessment. 2019;23(60):1–88.
20. Piegorsch WW. Sample sizes for improved binomial confidence intervals. Computational Statistics & Data Analysis. 2004;46(2):309–16.
21. Hampson LV, Whitehead J, Eleftheriou D, Tudur-Smith C, Jones R, Jayne D, et al. Elicitation of expert prior opinion: application to the MYPAN trial in childhood polyarteritis nodosa. PLoS One. 2015;10(3):e0120981.
22. Zheng H, Hampson LV. A Bayesian decision-theoretic approach to incorporate preclinical information into phase I oncology trials. Biometrical Journal. Biometrische Zeitschrift. 2020;62(6):1408–27.
23. Spiegelhalter DJ, Abrams KR, Myles JP. Bayesian Approaches to Clinical Trials and Health-Care Evaluation. Chichester: John Wiley & Sons; 2004.

6

Setting up a clinical trial

> The recruitment processes of an RCT should be carefully planned and piloted regardless of size or complexity.
>
> **Barbara Farrell and colleagues, 2010 (1)**

A complex web of processes and forms

Clinical trials are complex, multidisciplinary projects that integrate science, ethics, and legal requirements in the conduct of healthcare research. Careful planning and set-up are fundamental to the successful conduct of the study. Furthermore, setting up a trial within legal regulations, abiding by institutional policies and according to international standards (e.g. GCP (2)), is demanding and will require careful oversight in order to keep the study on track.

Regulations and related processes vary over time, sometimes even year to year, and certainly between countries. The specifics of legal acts and associated regulations, and related language will be avoided in this chapter as far as possible except where necessary or of key importance. Reference will be made predominantly to the UK setting with some key differences in the US and elsewhere noted. For the UK setting, it should be noted that currently the regulations are very similar to those of countries in the EU. However, the full impact of Brexit is yet to work through the system and aspects of the regulations may be more fluid over the next 5–10 years than perhaps has ever previously been the case. Similarly, the impact of the COVID-19 pandemic has affected clinical trial regulations and processes as it has done in other areas of life. It has led to a number of changes in practices and expectations. Most pertinently, there is greater acceptance of solely electronic documentation and more flexible implementation of some requirements (e.g. monitoring of study centres). It remains to be seen how much this translates into permanent changes in approach or if it is more a hiatus before returning to prior practices.

In this chapter we will consider the role of sponsorship of the clinical trial, and the approvals that may be needed to conduct the trial. We will also consider the critical nature of the type of clinical trial in determining the required approvals, the importance of ethical review of the clinical trial, and key documentation required for approval along with setting up centres. Finally, the process of developing and finalizing the protocol will be considered along with some of the key decisions that will have to be made as part of that process. This chapter will necessarily introduce a lot of terminology which must be confronted particularly for conducting trials that evaluate drugs. Indeed, even here right at the beginning we are confronted with new terminology as the UK (and EU) legislation refers to a 'investigational medicinal product' (IMP) not a 'drug'. However, as far as possible the use of terminology is kept to a minimum. Where the term IMP is used it indicates a drug treatment that falls within the UK (and EU) regulations. The use of 'drug' refers to the type of treatment and does not per se indicate whether it would be considered an IMP or not (though typically it would be). Reference to specifics of the system in many countries is not possible as, regrettably, many similar though slightly different terms and processes are often used for essentially the same thing. To give a taste of the scope of the challenge to be confronted when setting up a clinical trial, a summary of the stages in setting up and conducting of a clinical trial is given in Figure 6.1. Once the research question, objectives, PICOTS, and basic outline of a clinical trial design has been developed, a key early and critical step is confirmation of who will act as the sponsor of the clinical trial.

Sponsorship

The sponsor of a research project is an individual, company, institution, or any other organization or group that oversees the study from beginning to end. In short, the sponsor is the one who is held legally accountable for any issues that may arise. The sponsor must ensure proper arrangements are in place to initiate, conduct, and report the research study. In many countries this is an explicit legal requirement. All clinical trials of IMPs (CTIMPs for short) in the UK (3) are legally required to have a sponsor. Other types of clinical trials (e.g. a clinical trial of two types of surgery) would be expected to have one as well given they involve human participants and their healthcare, and the collection of data. As sponsorship results in hefty obligations on the sponsor, it is typically only institutions such as hospitals, universities, and medium to large companies that will act as the sponsor of a clinical trial. Indeed, it is possible for multiple entities to share the role of sponsor either by jointly sharing in all aspects or dividing up the responsibilities between themselves (3). The sponsor may be the company that developed a drug, or medical device, or the institution within which a new drug has been developed. In an academic

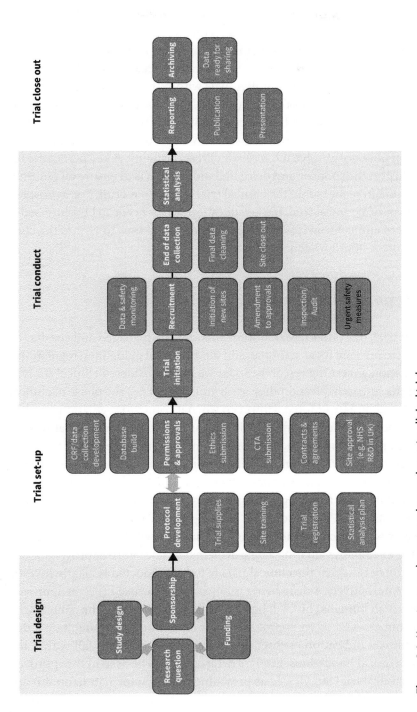

Figure 6.1 Key stages and processes in carrying out a clinical trial.
Note: R&D, research and development.

setting, it is typically the institution to which the prospective chief investigator (lead researcher) of the trial belongs that takes on the sponsorship role. The chief investigator is the named individual who is the lead for the study and accountable for it. The sponsor will typically delegate onwards to another institution, company, group, or individuals within the sponsoring institution specific responsibilities in order that it fulfils its duties. These responsibilities in turn may be delegated to specific individuals but ultimately responsibility lies in a practical sense with the chief investigator and the research team. Delegation does not absolve the sponsor of responsibility. A key part of the responsibility on the sponsor and delegated individuals is to ensure all required approvals are in place before the clinical trial begins to recruit. For a prospective sponsor of a clinical trial, the key question which needs to be addressed is what type of clinical trial it is, in order to understand how to ensure the clinical trial can be appropriately conducted.

What type of clinical trial is it?

A clinical trial, like other research studies, should be managed and conducted according to relevant local, national, and international guidelines, regulations, and legislation governing research. So far we have considered clinical trials in terms of the research question they are trying to address, the phase of clinical trial, and trial design adopted. However, when it comes to regulations the key categorization is rather disparate with substantially different implications for setting-up and conducting the trial depending upon the type.

The first and most important key question in this context is whether the clinical trial is evaluating an IMP or not (4). To be an IMP, it obviously needs to be a medicinal product (or 'drug' in common language). However, not all drug trials are trials of IMPs. The adjective 'investigational' refers to evaluating it in a particular way which means the clinical trial falls within the relevant legislation. For example, evaluating a new drug that has not been approved for use in the country in which the clinical trial is to be conducted is clearly investigational. Alternatively, a drug being used could be licensed (i.e. an approved drug for use in humans) but will be used in a different way in the clinical trial which is not covered by its approval. An example would be using it on a different ('clinical indication') subset of patients which does not fall within the approved clinical indications. Lastly, a drug could still be used in the approved way in a clinical trial but viewed as providing further information on this approval so as to still fall within the legislation. In short, clinical trials of drugs are likely to fall within the legislation and be classed as a CTIMP in the UK and the EU similarly. This is true even if the drug has been approved for medical use in humans, though only the relevant body (e.g. the MHRA in the UK) can give the final confirmation of this.

In different countries slightly different language is used for in essence the same thing, and the regulations may have slightly different coverage. In the US the corresponding terminology for an IMP is an 'investigational new drug' (IND) (5,6). In many countries it is a criminal offence to conduct a clinical trial of an IMP, IND, or equivalent without authorization from a specified body. In the UK, it is the MHRA who takes on this role and which grants authorization. In the US and Canada, it is the FDA and Health Canada, respectively, who undertake this authorization role. In the EU, it can be any one of the designated bodies in the member states (e.g. L'Agence nationale de sécurité du médicament et des produits de santé (ANSM) in France) who authorize the conduct of a clinical trial of drug treatments. Elsewhere in the world there may be a similar body (such as the Drug Controller General of India (DCGI) in India). Aside from authorization of the clinical trial, there may be separate regulations about how the clinical trial should be conducted. For example, in the EU it is the European Medicines Agency (EMA) that makes the recommendations about approval of drugs for medical use. Even though the authorization of clinical trials occurs at the national (EU member state) level, the EMA plays a key role in ensuring the standards of GCP are applied (2). Interestingly, many of the expectations for the conduct of the studies to be submitted within an authorization application to the EMA apply irrespective of whether the clinical trials are conducted within the EU or not. It is mandatory for information on the protocol and results of a clinical trial of an IMP that has received clinical trial authorization (CTA) to be posted on the EudraCT database (7) if the clinical trial is conducted in the EU or the European Economic Area (and irrespective of where it was conducted if it relates to a paediatric submission). Select information is then posted on the EU Clinical Trials Register (8) (except for phase 1 trials in adults), making this information publicly available. It is worth noting that the ICH has done excellent work to bring more harmony and consistency in approach across jurisdictions. It provides guidance about many aspects of conducting a clinical trial of an IMP including how to identify a medicinal product (9). Many of the documents are of great value, if not directly relevant to other (non-IMP) clinical trials.

The second related key question to consider when setting up a clinical trial is whether the clinical trial is evaluating a medical device or not. One might be tempted to say that answering the first question resolves the second, but alas the world of regulations is not necessarily that straightforward. To add to the confusion, trials of medical devices have in many countries their own specific, and substantially different, regulatory requirements. In terms of the legislation, it tends to require a clear interpretation of the intervention and control under evaluation as either a medical device or an IMP, or neither, to know what is required. Ultimately this may need the relevant body to confirm the investigators' view is correct unless it is completely clear. On the face of it this seems not too onerous though a number of drug treatments require invasive medical devices to deliver the IMP (e.g. drug eluding stents). In contrast, if we consider the TOPKAT trial which compared two types of knee surgery (see Chapter 2), it is clearly not a CTIMP or drug trial of any kind (10). However, is it a medical device trial? The research question posed is seeking to compare the treatments not specific devices per se which suggests it is not seeking (scientifically) to compare the medical devices. However, it could be a medical device trial under the UK, Canadian, EU, and US regulations. This depends upon whether devices to be used in the clinical trial have been approved or not for use, and whether the data from the trial might form a submission to obtain approval for use of an unapproved device, and the nature of the device (e.g. in Canada approval is only needed for some types of devices). The TOPKAT trial fortunately did not require any additional regulatory notification related to the medical devices used as they were already approved and in clinical use as per their use in the trial. Overall, the requirements for IMPs are much more onerous than for medical devices. Many medical devices will be approved on the basis of clinical data relating to another ('similar') device. Devices may be classified accordingly to perceived risk and requirement for approval vary accordingly. In the UK and the EU these are classes as I, IIa, IIb, and III; the higher the classification, the more 'risky' the device is perceived and the greater scrutiny, in principle at least, the approval of the device receives. A key feature of the classification is whether it is 'implantable', that is, a medical device which is introduced by surgical procedure into the body, whether completely or partially, which is intended to remain there (e.g. a pacemaker that is inserted and left within the body). Another key feature in determining the classification is whether it is 'active' or not, that is, a medical device with a power source (e.g. a pacemaker would be considered as such but a typical knee implant would not).

If a clinical trial involving a medical device which does not have regulatory approval for use is planned, this will typically require notification in advance of starting the study (11). For example, in the UK, it is currently necessary to notify the MHRA 60 days before initiating such a study. In the US, an investigational device exemption (12) will be required before the clinical trial of a medical device without marketing authorization can proceed. The notification packet for such approvals will require substantial documentation relating to the device, its development, and its manufacturing, along with information on the 'clinical investigation' (i.e. the clinical trial) planned including details on the management and investigators. During the notification period the safety and performance of the medical device will be assessed along with the design of the clinical investigation. A notification will be received about whether an objection or not has been raised to the conducting of the study. Raised objections tend to be related to demonstrating the safety or technical effectiveness of the device though the design of the clinical investigation may also be questioned. While post-marketing surveillance of some kind will be required for devices, this will typically fall far short of the scientific standards that clinical trials seek to adhere to. The studies tend to be passive, and incomplete, and pick up mostly on the more obvious and severe device-related safety events.

The third question to ask is whether the trial falls under any special remit requiring special approvals. An example of a special approval is requiring an exception for the purpose of the trial for transfer of confidential patient information without consent (Confidentiality Advisory Group section 251 approval in the UK). Another area for additional approval is the use of a radioactive substance in a clinical trial which requires certification from the Administration of Radioactive Substances Advisory Committee in the UK. Similarly, use of gene therapy is treated as a special case and requires review by a specific national research ethics committee (REC). Conveniently for those conducting clinical trials in the UK, the whole process is handled to a large extent by a single system called the Integrated Research Application System (IRAS) (13).

The fourth question to ask is whether the clinical trial or aspects of its conduct fall under addition regulations. Examples include the additional requirements to ensure appropriate handling of recruitment where children are involved, and recruiting individuals who do not have the capacity to consent. For the latter, a process to address and later request consent if capacity is regained is normally expected. Of note, the loss of capacity of a participant after consenting also has implications for all clinical trials in the UK. Another aspect where additional regulations apply is the transportation of infectious or dangerous samples which might be undertaken in a clinical trial (e.g. participant samples for COVID-19 polymerase chain reaction testing). Similarly, the handling of data and in particular the transfer of data between organizations will fall under the corresponding data protection and privacy laws. In the UK, the Data Protection Act 2018 and EU General Data Protection Regulation (GDPR) apply, the latter as tailored to the UK. Collectively the requirements are referred to as the 'UK GDPR' (14). See the following sections for further consideration of data-related issues and Table 6.1 for a summary of the key questions to ask to determine the type of clinical trial.

Table 6.1 Key questions to ask to determine the clinical trial type (UK context)

Question	Implications
Is it a clinical trial evaluating an investigational medicinal product (15)?	• *Specific legal framework and regulations may apply* (e.g. Medicines for Human Use (Clinical Trials) Regulations 2004 (SI 2004/1031 in the UK)) (3,4). Some non-IMP medicinal products fall under separate regulations (e.g. unlicensed medicinal products specifically manufactured in accordance with authorized health professional for use in individual patients under their care: 'specials') (16) • *Special approval is needed prior to initiation* (e.g. CTA approval from the MHRA) (4) • *International standard may apply* (ICH guidelines (17) relating to quality, efficacy, safety, and multidisciplinary topics) • *Additional registration and reporting requirement may apply* (e.g. registering the trial, or entering protocol info on EUDRACT) (7)
Does the clinical trial evaluate a medical device?	• *Specific legal frameworks may apply* (e.g. in the UK, the Medical Devices Regulations 2002 (11)) • *Special approval may be needed prior to initiation* (e.g. the clinical investigation plan along with related documents (such as the details of the device, consent form, etc.) need to be submitted and there needs to be no objection raised by the MHRA (unless the medical device is covered by marketing approval for the purpose it is being used for in the clinical trial)) (11) • *Relevant international standards may apply* even if not legally required (18)
Are additional approvals required?	• Does the clinical trial involve the *use of human tissue* (a specific licence may be needed by the relevant institutions involved)? (19) • Is a *gene therapy* involved? Clinical trials involving a gene therapy require approval from the Gene Therapy Advisory Committee (a national REC for gene therapy clinical research) (20) • Is a radioactive substance being used? Approval is needed for the administration of a radioactive substantive (21)
Are additional regulations invoked by the clinical trial procedures?	• Does the trial *recruit children and young people*? Legal recognition of capacity to consent will vary between legal jurisdictions, and according to the type of study (22). In the UK, a minimum of 16 years of age is needed to be considered an adult and have the clear right to give legal consent without reference to a parent or legal guardian. The position of those aged 16 or 17 years but not yet 18 years of age varies accordingly to the individual's capacity in England, Wales, and Northern Ireland and whether the clinical trial is a CTIMP or not. In Scotland, 16 years is the legal age of consent. Those under 16 may in some circumstance be considered able to consent if they are deemed to have competency but not for CTIMPs • Will any of the potential participants *lack capacity* at the time of recruitment? Are they likely to lose capacity during the clinical trial? In these circumstances additional legislative requirements may be invoked. In specific circumstances an individual may be entered into a trial prior to legal consent being obtained. Aside from legal requirements, the views of children and parents or legal guardians should be considered where relevant

Obtaining ethical approval

A universal principle and expectation to ensure safety of patients and protection of their rights is an independent ethical review of the proposed study (e.g. a clinical trial) prior to commencement. Typically this is done by a body with a specific remit to undertake such an ethical review of research studies. Such a body is according to the FDA regulations 'to review, approve the initiation of and conduct periodic review of biomedical research involving human subjects'. The primary purpose of such a review is to 'ensure the protection of the rights and welfare of the human subject' (23). This ethical review body should be made up of individuals with various backgrounds (scientific specialisms, members of the public, and others) who will typically be volunteers. Membership of such a committee is often a substantial time commitment for which there is often no direct compensation. Each body will have their own policies and processes about how the review process will proceed. US government-funded research is required to follow the 'Common Rule' which are the federal regulations that are based upon the 'Belmont Report'. This report was produced in 1978 and summarizes ethical principles and guidelines for research involving human subjects. The three fundamental ethical principles for any research that involves human subjects are respect for persons, beneficence, and justice. Many US academic institutions require their staff to uphold these standards irrespective of funding (24). For a body to be considered to be a 'duly constituted institutional review board' for conducting the ethical reviews, it may need to follow specific regulations about its formation (e.g. membership of the committee) and its operation (having a majority of its membership present at the review meeting) (25). A booking may well be required to ensure a slot is available when the ethical review is desired. Specific documentation will have to be submitted in advance and a small number of members of the ethics review body may be specifically delegated the task of undertaking an initial review on behalf of the group prior to a full meeting. In particular, the review body will require seeing the protocol of the study, and any documentation which will be viewed by prospective or actual participants. Expedited review where initiation of the trial is particularly time sensitive (e.g. a COVID-19 treatment trial) may be possible to speed up the review process. Proportionate review (i.e. reduced level of scrutiny) might also be available, though clinical trials are unlikely to fall within the corresponding criteria.

Of key interest to the ethics committee will be the process of consenting to participate in the study (or assenting on behalf of those unable to do so for themselves, e.g. for children or adults with capacity). Accordingly, the information provided at the point at which the prospective participant (or their representative) is introduced to the study is critically important, as well as the consent form through which the consent for an individual's participation is recorded. Similarly, the information collected directly from the participant and the processes in place to protect the rights of participants and their data will be of key interest. Trials typically have a patient information leaflet which is provided to the prospective participant to explain in accessible language what the study is about, why it is being carried out, what participation will be required, and the rights of the individual to decline or cease participation at any point. A representative of the investigators may be allowed to attend or participate in part of the corresponding review meeting to answer questions, and to clarify aspects of the study proposal. The proposed study will be assessed regarding the safety implications for participants in terms of the benefits and risks to them, and the process by which individuals may be recruited to the study. Furthermore, it is generally accepted that while the scientific quality of the study is not in the committee's remit, to be 'ethical', a study must be scientifically valid. Each study reviewed will receive an 'ethical opinion' about it and whether it should go ahead, and, if so, whether any conditions should be applied. It is not uncommon for conditions to impact the scientific design of the study even though this is not the primary focus of the ethical review. Appealing a decision may be possible if the initial outcome is 'unfavourable' and considered by the investigators to be inappropriate, though grounds for the appeal will be needed.

Different names are used for a group essentially carrying out the same task, such as an ethical review board, REC, or institutional review board. Sponsors will have different expectations about the appropriate body for the clinical trials they sponsor. Review by a specific body may be mandatory due to the setting in which the study is taking place. For example, any clinical trial recruiting individuals from NHS services in the UK will be required to be reviewed by the National (UK Health Departments) Research Ethics Service. The review is undertaken by one of the related RECs, and a single submission covers all centres (within the UK NHS). Any CTIMP or medical device trial (i.e. a clinical investigation of a medical device) must similarly be legally reviewed. As such, almost all clinical trials conducted in the UK will be legally required to be ethically reviewed. Even if not strictly legally required for all, this must still be the expectation. There is no reason to expect any less in other countries even if legally it is not enforced.

For most clinical trials, achieving a favourable ethical opinion might be seen to be in little doubt. While few could reasonably doubt the value of an 'independent' ethical review, the process can be somewhat daunting, time-consuming, and frustrating. The great ethical principle of protecting participants' rights can become a somewhat bureaucratic process which investigators need to negotiate. Nevertheless, as we saw in Chapter 1, history regrettably demonstrates to us the need for legal boundaries to protect individuals' rights (including in clinical trials). As such, ethical reviews need to be viewed by investigators as a key part of a healthy research process. While not 'infallible', submitting to the process demonstrates the intention to carry out research that follows GCP by the investigators (and sponsor) aside from the legal requirement. Sometimes the review will identify a problem prior to study initiation, perhaps even of a critical nature, which will enable the investigators to address it prior to commencement of recruitment.

Following data protection laws

Data protection laws also have an important impact upon the design and set-up of clinical trials. Sponsors and ethical review bodies will look to see that appropriate legislation is referred to and accounted for in the clinical trial processes. In particular, they will scrutinize the patient consent process and the handling and retention of data. This area is particularly challenging for clinical trials which will be conducted across multiple countries. All the respective legislation will need to be considered when formulating the approaches adopted in the clinical trial. Data sharing agreements will be needed between entities which can be time-consuming to secure, and can lead to length delays, particularly across country borders (and correspondingly in and out of the EU).

In the UK, the key law regarding data is the Data Protection Act 2018, which replaced the earlier Data Protection Act 1998. This legislation translated the EU GDPR into UK law, and instituted the UK GDPR (14). These laws restrict the processing of personal data and require a legal basis for this activity. The key point to note is that medical data are classified as personal data. The legislation clearly specifies that personal data will need to be processed in a particular and more restrictive way. Clinical trials clearly involve the 'processing' of personal data and therefore need to reflect the requirements. Furthermore, some data collected in clinical trials will be designated as being 'special category data'. This is personal data that is viewed as particularly sensitive (e.g. information on genetic information, health, and sex life). To process personal data there must be a legal basis for its use, and in the case of special category data additional stipulations apply regarding the legal basis. Overall, the basis of using personal data may be to meet other legal obligations such as safety reporting related to IMP use. It could also be to carry out a task in the public interest, one under the legitimate interest of the controller, one to be carried out upon scientific grounds, or with the data subject's (i.e. the trial participant and any associated individuals for whom data is to be collected) explicit consent. This consent to use of personal data should not be confused with 'informed consent' to participate in the clinical trial which cannot be used as a 'catch all' consent for all activities from a data protection point of view. Therefore, clinical trial consent forms will typically have specific consents relevant to the processing of data, and particularly regarding data transfer to third parties.

Under the legislation it is important to define the data controller and data processors. The data controller (i.e. the sponsor, lead institution, and/or investigators) has the obligation to ensure the data is processed accordingly. Data processors (those who process the data) act only under the authority of the data controller. If data can be anonymized (i.e. it is no longer possible to identify the subject), it will no longer be considered personal data under the GDPR. However, only at the very end of a trial, and even then, only in a limited way, could clinical trial data be rendered fully anonymized prior to use without markedly diluting its quality. Unfortunately, the GDPR has in many ways produced less clarity in terms of data protection requirement for clinical trials as is the case for other types of clinical research. Furthermore, different bodies applying essentially the same principles may come to a different conclusion about what is and what is not covered. Therefore, explicit consent for data processing (including collecting, and sharing data with other parties) is warranted whenever possible in addition to the application of any other legal basis, in order to be confident of the legal basis at the present time.

Investigational medicinal product clinical trial approval documentation

Obtaining specific approval for conducting a clinical trial of an IMP is required in many countries such as the UK, the US, and EU member states among others. Securing this approval requires along with perhaps the obvious clinical trial documents (e.g. trial protocol, care report forms, consent form, etc.), a number of other documents as part of the submission process. The key ones for an application to conduct a CTIMP in the UK (and EU) will be considered briefly below. Permission for this is called a CTA.

Investigator's brochure

The investigator's brochure is a document that details the clinical and non-clinical data on the investigational products to be used in the clinical trial (17). The aim is to provide the investigators delivering the trial with the relevant information to understand the clinical processes related to the IMP use and safety monitoring processes. It should also allow them to assess the potential benefits and risks entailed in participation in the clinical trial. Additionally, it can provide information useful for the clinical management of individual patients involved in the clinical trial. The investigator's brochure may require updating when additional relevant information becomes available (e.g. the findings from a new study using the IMP). Details included should relate to the specifics of non-clinical studies, pharmacological (PK and PD) properties in animals, along with a summary of the effect of the IMP in humans covering pharmacological (PK and PD) properties and safety and efficacy information (e.g. dose–response relationship).

Investigational medicinal product dossier

An IMP dossier is a document required to conduct a clinical trial of an IMP in the UK and the EU. This document summarizes information on the quality, manufacture, and control of the IMP as it will be used in the clinical trial (26). Typically, testing of the properties of the IMP are required in order to receive authorization for use in humans via a CTA application. What is required will vary according to the IMP development to date (i.e. phase of clinical trial to be undertaken). Where the IMP has marketing authorization and is being used in the same form for a covered indication and dose regimen, the summary of product characteristics (SmPC) may suffice instead of a separate IMP dossier.

Summary of product characteristics

For IMPs with marketing authorization, a SmPC (27) is included as part of the CTA application which will be used if the clinical trial is approved. The SmPC provides all details required to be able to use the IMP in clinical practice including its brand name, composition and quantity of each active ingredient, form (e.g. tablet), clinical parameters, details on how it should be used or taken, pharmacological properties (PK and PD), preclinical safety data, and pharmaceutical properties (e.g. storage and shelf life), among other things.

Manufacturing and import authorization

Documentation related to ensuring compliance with good manufacturing practice is also required as part of the CTA application. A UK site wishing to manufacture or assemble an IMP requires the manufacturer's authorization. The corresponding documentation is called a MIA(IMP) (manufacturing and import authorization for an IMP). In EU countries an alternative licence is required. Where an IMP is not manufactured and authorized for use within the clinical trial host legal jurisdiction (e.g. UK or EU), importer authorization will also be required to be demonstrated to receive a CTA. At least one 'qualified person' (QP) will need to be named in the licence who is responsible for ensuring every batch of the medicinal product has been manufactured and/or assembled and checked in accordance with legal requirements. To be the QP, an individual must meet specific professional requirements (e.g. a pharmacist who has membership of the Royal Pharmaceutical Society). In the UK there is an exemption (regulation 37) (3) for hospitals and health centres which do not require a specific MIA(IMP) for assembly (i.e. putting the manufactured IMP into a container, and/or labelling it for use in the clinical trial) of an IMP, if used in a clinical trial and carried out under supervision of doctor or pharmacist. The specific IMP to be used in the clinical trial must be certified by the QP before it can be release for use in the clinical trial (this is called 'QP release').

IMP label

The design of the clinical trial study drug label must be submitted to the relevant regulatory authority for assessment as part of the CTA. There are strict requirements for the information which is presented regarding the contact details for information on the product and clinical trial (e.g. if emergency unblinding is needed for a patient in a placebo-controlled trial), the name of the IMP (and placebo/comparator if a blinded trial), route of administration and dose (e.g. oral, one tablet twice daily), and clinical trial subject reference and/or trial subject identifier. An example of a labelled bottle containing an IMP for use in a regulated clinical trial is shown in Figure 6.2 (28).

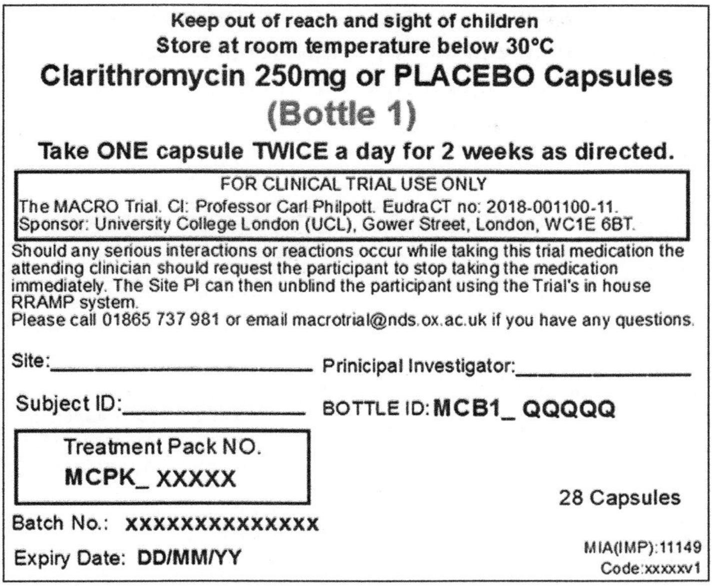

```
┌─────────────────────────────────────────────────────────────────────┐
│              Keep out of reach and sight of children                  │
│               Store at room temperature below 30°C                    │
│          Clarithromycin 250mg or PLACEBO Capsules                     │
│                          (Bottle 1)                                   │
│         Take ONE capsule TWICE a day for 2 weeks as directed.         │
│  ┌──────────────────────────────────────────────────────────────┐    │
│  │                 FOR CLINICAL TRIAL USE ONLY                    │    │
│  │ The MACRO Trial. CI: Professor Carl Philpott. EudraCT no: 2018-001100-11. │
│  │ Sponsor: University College London (UCL), Gower Street, London, WC1E 6BT. │
│  └──────────────────────────────────────────────────────────────┘    │
│  Should any serious interactions or reactions occur while taking this trial medication the │
│  attending clinician should request the participant to stop taking the medication │
│  immediately. The Site PI can then unblind the participant using the Trial's in house │
│  RRAMP system.                                                        │
│  Please call 01865 737 981 or email macrotrial@nds.ox.ac.uk if you have any questions. │
│                                                                       │
│  Site:_____ Prinicipal Investigator:_____    │
│                                                                       │
│  Subject ID:_____  BOTTLE ID: MCB1_ QQQQQ                  │
│  ┌────────────────────────────┐                                      │
│  │  Treatment Pack NO.         │                                      │
│  │   MCPK_ XXXXX               │                                      │
│  │                             │          28 Capsules                 │
│  └────────────────────────────┘                                      │
│  Batch No.:  XXXXXXXXXXXXXX                                           │
│  Expiry Date: DD/MM/YY                        MIA(IMP):11149          │
│                                               Code:xxxxxv1            │
└─────────────────────────────────────────────────────────────────────┘
```

Figure 6.2 IMP label design used in the MACRO trial (28).

Developing and finalizing the protocol

The receipt of approvals which we have considered in previous sections presumes the protocol for the clinical trial (or equivalently the 'clinical investigational plan' for medical device trials in the UK and EU) has been developed and finalized. In this section we consider some of the key aspects which will require further development and refinement as part of the process of producing a complete trial protocol ready for submission for approvals (sponsor, ethics, etc.). Having reached the point of setting up a clinical trial, the rough outline of the protocol will have been reviewed and refined and should be at the point where the research question the study is seeking to answer has been clearly thrashed out. Nevertheless, substantially more work is needed to turn a well-worked clinical trial proposal into an implementable protocol. The sponsor will often have a template for a protocol which they would like to be used. This may be specific to the study type (e.g. clinical trial of an IMP). Templates will vary in formats and heading and sections, some involving more repetition than others. Nevertheless, using such a template helps avoid unnecessary confusion as the sponsor's reviewer will be familiar with it and it will help prevent omission of key information. An example of the table of contents for a protocol is given in Figure 6.3. If this is compared to the SPIRIT (Standard Protocol Items: Recommendations for Interventional Trials) (29) checklist of 33 items for reporting in protocols, one can readily see many of the same items appearing. See Chapter 10 for consideration of reporting standards like

STUDY PERSONNEL AND CONTACT DETAILS	SAFETY EVENTS AND REPORTING
SYNOPSIS	Definitions
ABBREVIATIONS	Causality
STUDY BACKGROUND AND RATIONALE	Study treatment related serious adverse events
Background	Reporting of events
Rationale	Protocol deviations
STUDY OBJECTIVES AND PURPOSE	Serious breaches
Purpose	**ETHICAL AND REGULATORY ASPECTS**
Primary objective	Ethics committee and regulatory approvals
Secondary objectives	Informed consent and participant Information
STUDY DESIGN	Study documentation
Primary outcome	Case report forms
Secondary outcomes	Sample labelling
Safety outcomes	Source documents
Stopping rules and discontinuation	Data protection
Randomisation and blinding	Record retention and archiving
Handling of randomisation codes and procedures for unblinding	Discontinuation of the study
STUDY MANAGEMENT	**QUALITY ASSURANCE AND AUDIT**
Study committees	Risk assessment
Data monitoring and safety committee	Study monitoring
Trial steering committee	Quality assurance
Trial management group	Insurance and indemnity
Study duration	Study conduct
Participant involvement	Reporting
End of the study	**USER AND PUBLIC INVOLVEMENT**
RECRUITMENT AND WITHDRAWAL OF PARTICIPANTS	**STUDY FINANCES**
Recruitment process	Funding
Eligibility criteria	Participant payments
Discontinuation of treatments or assessments	**ARCHIVING**
STUDY TREATMENTS	**REFERENCES**
Treatment descriptions	**APPENDIX-PUBLICATION AND DISSEMINATION POLICY**
Adherence	
Criteria for terminating study	
Transport and storage of the blood samples	
Laboratory analyses	
STATISTICAL METHODOLOGY	
Statistical analysis plan	
Approach and methods	
Timing of analyses	
Sample size and justification	
Decision points	
Stopping rules	

Figure 6.3 Table of contents of protocol for a CTIMP.

SPIRIT. However, it is worth noting that a protocol that is approvable by a sponsor will have more information on less academic but ethically and regulatory important topics. Such topics include data auditing, safety monitoring processes, and archiving of study data and documentation once the clinical trial closes. Furthermore, a sponsor may also have standard text applicable to their setting (or the typical settings for the clinical trials they sponsor). There has been a big shift in expectations for such aspects and how detailed protocols should be over the last 30 years. The core protocol for the International Stroke Trial (IST) (30) conducted in the 1990s was only 24 pages long and included key trial documents. Protocols stretching to over 100 pages are not unheard of these days. If all protocol-related documents are included such as information sheets, consent forms, and data collection forms, we could easily be talking about a few hundred pages for some clinical trials.

Having access to the approval protocol from a previously approved clinical trial can help save a lot of time when developing a protocol for a new clinical trial. There is the danger of ignorantly cutting and pasting which cannot be over-emphasized. Clinical trial protocols are complex and trial specific. All elements need to be considered in light of each other to ensure they make sense, are appropriate, and are implementable. Similarly, clear document control is vital as is review by all the key members of the investigator team and other relevant areas of expertise. Prior to confirmation of sponsorship, the sponsor will expect to be able to review a draft protocol in advance of review by regulatory bodies (e.g. ethical review boards or regulatory agencies such as the MHRA or the FDA). We consider below five key aspects of the clinical trial protocol: confirming the trial population, defining the trial treatments, scheduling trial follow-up and assessment, defining the trial outcomes, and safety data collection and reporting.

Key decisions in developing and finalizing the protocol

Trial population

A key step in moving from a trial proposal to an implementable protocol is clarifying the population of interest. The broad group of interest should by now be clear but in terms of implementing the protocol, an actionable set of criteria needs to be presented. This is typically done by identifying in the 'inclusion criteria' the general group of individuals (e.g. patients) of interest. A list of exclusion criteria is then used to exclude individuals from the inclusion criteria (i.e. individuals who met the inclusion criteria but who are thought not appropriate to take part in the study). A very common example is the exclusion, not always for good reasons, of pregnant women from being eligible to take part in a study even though they are otherwise suitable (i.e. met the inclusion criteria). If we return to the TOPKAT trial example, our main group of interest are patients with medial osteoarthritis of the knee (10). To be able to first identify this group we need to clarify the age range. For example, is it adults only, and if so, what is the youngest age we would be interested in, is it 16 or 18 years old? While osteoarthritis of the knee tends to be age related in that it is usually caused by wear and tear (e.g. older age and at least 40 years old) there can be rare exceptions where children get the disease. Therefore, we might insist upon participants being at least 16 years of age. This would also have the benefit of simplifying the consent process (even more so if we move to 18 years and above for the UK). It might seem clinically obvious that we would not include anyone younger than this to a surgeon and other medical professionals. However, it is important that the protocol is explicit in who is potentially eligible for the study. Furthermore, we also need to consider what we mean by someone having medial osteoarthritis of the knee. Ultimately, we are looking for someone with clinically diagnosed disease but we could accept *any* existing clinical diagnosis of medial knee osteoarthritis. Alternatively, we could stipulate that a particular test or tests have been part of the diagnosis (e.g. computed tomography or MRI scan assessment). Or we could require an additional scan as part of the eligibility process for the clinical trial (again with varying degrees of specificity in testing modalities) and the diagnosis process (local doctor and/or centralized confirmation). Furthermore, we could also specify the period for which the patient has had a clinical diagnosis of medial knee osteoarthritis. Another consideration is about related physiology of the knee and whether restrictions are needed (e.g. is only isolated medial osteoarthritis acceptable?). As the comparison is between partial and total knee replacement this would seem a natural choice. Other choices relate to the general condition of the knee, with choices to be made about stipulations regarding the state of the knee cartilage and ligaments. Finally, there needs to be a decision about whether a clinical assessment (local or centralized) of suitability for surgery and/or basic fitness criteria for surgery (American Society of Anesthesiologists grade of 1 or 2, i.e. otherwise healthy patient or at most has only a mild systemic disease) will be required. These choices all have implications for the recruitment of patients. They affect the number who will meet the criteria, and the timing of when potential patients will need to be approached in their care pathway. They also affect the practicality of implementing the recruitment strategy at various centres which may have rather different systems for the care of patients.

Having defined the inclusion population, we turn our attention to the exclusion criteria. We could also think about what prior treatment individuals need to have had prior to participating in the clinical trial. If someone has had prior surgery on the knee, are they suitable to take part in the clinical trial? As revision surgery is generally considered to be substantially more difficult than primary surgery, we might wish to exclude such patients. Injury to the other (lateral) side of the knee might also be considered an exclusion to having a partial knee replacement and therefore might be excluded. Other common areas of exclusion are those individuals who have related and complicated conditions, such as other types of arthritis or inflammatory diseases, or problems with their foot, hip or spine that make assessment of the knee challenging. Finally, we might wish to exclude those who for various reasons may not be likely to fulfil the required commitments of participation in the study (e.g. visits to the hospital due to residential location, inability to complete questionnaires, etc.). All of these exclusions can be reasonable, as are potentially others. However, each additional criterion makes the eligibility assessment process more complicated, time-consuming, and also reduces the pool of potential participants available to recruit to the study. Some specific requirements have a greater impact than others and as far as possible this should be assessed upfront. For other types of treatments, a similar process to the above will need to be undertaken. IMPs or other drugs will often have other drugs or substances with which they are known to work less well with or might lead to an increased risk of an adverse event (i.e. there are 'contraindications'). For example, simvastatin, a statin drug taken to lower cholesterol levels in the blood, interacts with grapefruit juice, thereby increasing the level of the drug in the blood (31,32). It is also common to exclude those who have previously received the drug being evaluated in the trial (if it is already available for medical use). Use of another drug that acts in the same way might also exclude individuals for a period thought to be sufficient to allow its effect to fully dissipate. This might cover both prior to and (as far is clinically appropriate) during the clinical trial. For each IMP or drug, careful consideration is needed of what is known about it and whether there are individuals, otherwise suitable for participation, who should not be involved. In general, the exclusions will reduce as the phase of the trial increases from 1 to 3; the exception being phase 1 first-in-human trials which may have health volunteers so potentially representing a large proportion of society. Phase 1 and 2 trials of efficacy often have fairly strict inclusion criteria. The phase 3 trial typically has a much broader, more inclusive population, preferably reflective, at least in part of potential clinical practice and use (current or future use if an IMP that is currently unlicensed is used beyond approved indications). Needless to say, the more narrow the focus on the inclusion and exclusion criteria, the less direct applicability the findings of the clinical trials will likely have.

Treatment definitions

The approach to defining the intervention and control will vary according to the type of treatment (e.g. drug versus surgery) and trial (CTIMP versus other drug-like products, e.g. vitamin and food supplements). An additional level of detail will likely be required for a protocol over a trial proposal in terms of how the intervention and control will be delivered. We will briefly define the treatments according to different treatment types.

IMP and other drug treatments

For an IMP (and any placebo or alternative IMP used within the trial), the protocol will need to provide explicit details about what it contains, the form it comes in, and how it is to be given to the participants. This will have to reflect the study design, and for a dose-escalation study or one with different does potentially given to participants, the process of determining which dose and how it is delivered needs to be clearly specified. The dose level to be used in a new participant may be based upon the occurrence of toxicity adverse events observed in previously recruited participants. The protocol should also clearly state the source of the IMP, its manufacture, distribution, and storage requirements, and reference as appropriate a MIA(IMP) and other relevant documents (such as SmPC, investigator's brochure, IMP dossier, etc.). The responsibilities related to ensuring the safe and secure storage and use of the IMP across different centres will need to be clearly stated. Typically this would be the responsibility of the centre's principal investigator (PI). This individual is the lead researcher on the study at the centre though they may delegate the responsibility regarding storage and use of the IMP to a pharmacist at the local centre, or equivalently qualified individual. How such delegation of duties will be recorded must be stated including use of a log or alternative. Furthermore, clear statements on the shipping arrangements need to be provided or reference made to a document which does (e.g. a summary of drug arrangements). The process of dispatching an IMP, and how replacement IMPs would be provided need to be clarified. In addition, the responsibility for monitoring the storage to ensure it is appropriate, and how any unused IMP will be disposed of, needs to be considered. Monitoring processes for use (where applicable, e.g. if participants are provided tablets or injections to take at home) should be stated. If a placebo is being used (or the product is not likely to be identifiable to participants or health professionals), a clear process for 'unblinding', that is, revealing the treatment received by a participant for an emergency situation, will be required. This needs to be readily available at any point during the trial as and when required. However, it also needs to be done in a way so as to record what was done. Additionally, it should not 'unblind' more than is strictly necessary to avoid undermining this aspect of the trial design beyond what is required. The potential need to 'unblind' will vary greatly according to the IMP, the population on which it is being used, and the phase of trial. The protocol needs to reference the approach and relevant documentation. As far as possible using centre-specific names and details should be avoided in detailing processes to ensure the set-up is implementable across multiple research centres, and to avoid requiring modification due to the procedures and infrastructure of specific centres. Finally, the process of participant care and how it relates to standard care following the completion of the treatment needs to be clearly stated to ensure patient safety and prevent any gaps in clinical oversight.

For other drug (but not IMP) treatments, the same general approach as above will be needed with similar specifics. If the drug is not considered an IMP some of the aforementioned documents may not be required. However, issues such as storage, handling, dispatch, and manufacture could still apply though conditions may be much less onerous and there may be much more flexibility about who handles what. Documentation of the key steps will still be needed and clearly specified in the protocol.

Non-drug treatments

Non-drug treatments come in a wonderful variety (33). In our examples we have already considered knee surgery but other notable examples include physiotherapy (physical therapy) and psychological treatments such as cognitive behaviour therapy, among others. The lack of adequate specification of these treatments in clinical trial protocols is common. While it is improving, this has been a consistently problematic area of conduct and reporting of clinical trials. To understand how bad it can be, we can consider an example trial which compared medical and surgical management provided in the trial report (published in a leading medical journal and for the time a well-conducted study): a single sentence stated that the surgery was either 'saphenous-vein graft or internal mammary artery' with no reference to the surgeon or setting (34). Two common distinctions between drug- and non-drug-based treatments are the importance of the deliverer, and the level of variability between instances of the treatment due to patient-related or operator preferences and choices. Fortunately, there are a number of helpful guides on evaluating and reporting these types of treatments, and relevant levels of specification (35–37). While strictly speaking a reporting guide (reporting being an aspect of clinical trials we will consider in more details in Chapter 10), the template for intervention description and replication (TIDieR) (38) checklist and guide, with its aim of improving replicability, is also a useful reference not only for trials of non-drug treatments, but also for drug trials (particularly of drugs with marketing approval). The latter sometimes similarly fail to clearly report the intervention and control in a way that makes clear what has been, and should be, done if one were to apply it in clinical practice.

Outcome specification

In Chapter 2 we considered briefly the outcome of primary outcome. However, for the protocol we need to provide a full list of outcomes to be collected and assessed. Returning to our knee surgery example, it is not enough to state the primary outcome will be patient-assessed pain and function, and provide a list of secondary outcomes of interest. We need to be explicit about how each outcome will be assessed. For example, in the TOPKAT trial (39), the primary outcome was the OKS, which is made up of 12 questions that are completed by patients, each with five levels of response. The final score ranges from 0 to 48 (each question response ranges from 0 to 4 and a higher response indicates a better response). When choosing specific tools or methods to assess the outcome, a number of aspects need to be considered. First, will it measure what is truly of interest? How reliable is the measurement? How readily can it be measured? Is any specific expertise or equipment required, and how easily can it be interpreted? In the OKS we have a questionnaire designed to be easily filled in by patients, that can be completed in about 5–10 minutes, has high completion rates, and has been shown to be reliable (40). Here we have considered the main aspects of interest, but there are increasingly extensive and elaborate approaches to assessing properties for questionnaire-based quality of life outcomes (41). In addition to the primary outcome, we will want to include a number of secondary outcomes. These need to cover both other benefits (positive effects) of the two operations and also any potential harms (negative effects). Reference should be made to any published core outcome set (set of outcome recommended to include in a phase 3 trial) for this clinical area to be included in clinical trials (42). Other types of knee assessments could be considered, including those which include more 'objective' assessments based upon range of motion, alignment, and stability of the knee in a quantitative sense (e.g. American Knee Society Score (43)). Complications arising from the operation and the need for further treatment, particularly surgery, will clearly be of interest. We might also want a more generic assessment of health such as the use of a EuroQol-5D questionnaire, perhaps the five-level version (44). All of the outcomes need to be clearly specified in the protocol in a way that can be implemented consistently and practically at all study centres. We will consider the associated data collection and monitoring in Chapter 7.

Scheduling trial follow-up and assessments

Having considered the population, the treatments and the outcomes in more detail we now need to think more about the scheduling of the follow-up and assessments. To ensure only appropriate individuals are included in a study, a process of screening is typically required prior to confirmation of eligibility and consenting prospective participants. Screening may require additional tests to be carried out. Any such tests and assessments will need to be scheduled and may well require an initial consent to screen prior to formally consenting an individual (i.e. asking an individual if they wish to take part in the study). For most studies recruitment happens over a sustained period of time and is carried out at research centres as potentially eligible participants are identified as part of routine medical care. Much less commonly, a pool of potential participants may already exist who can be approached almost simultaneously. Either way, the timing of any assessments need to be carefully planned according to how the potential participants are identified and approached. The timing of consent needs to be aligned so that all required checks of eligibility are completed and the results available, so that the consenting process can proceed.

Collection of key data on the participants needs to be planned for those who consent to take part (or for whom permission to participate is received), and who enter the study. The corresponding follow-up visits and assessment points need to be specified at the relevant time points. The scientifically optimal and most convenient way to conduct the follow-up is to have follow-up timed from the formal study entry (e.g. randomization in an RCT). This sets a consistent point in time for all participants. Baseline data is usually collected immediately on entry and prior to receipt of the treatments (and randomization if an RCT). There are, however, a number of practical constraints upon what follow-up can realistically be implemented and when. Participants will not typically be able, or wish, to regularly visit a healthcare centre if it is not linked to their general care. Research conducted around existing healthcare (e.g. most phase 3 trials) will be subsequently constrained by the availability of staff. Sufficient funding, which is mostly the preserve of trials sponsored and funded by commercial companies, may ease some structural constraints (e.g. providing for the use of exclusive facilities). However, there will still likely be restrictions on the availability of specialized staff (e.g. senior medical doctors) to undertake specific examinations. The follow-up schedules therefore need to be carefully considered for practicality and implementability, with more centres required typically leading to the need for more flexible and less onerous requirements. Related additional clinical care requirements (e.g. extra physiotherapy), even if adequately compensated, will have related pressures that may restrict the availability of tests, particularly those requiring specialized equipment and technical staff.

The pattern of follow-up needs to reflect the key research question the study is seeking to address though follow-up may in reality be a compromise between what is scientifically desirable and what can be achieved (at least in principle) for all patients. Therefore, the number and length of visits needs to be considered along with the time commitment and other obligations on the participants. For phase 1 trials recruiting health volunteers, substantial financial compensation is common given the expectation may be of, at least initially, hourly measurements continuing daily for perhaps a few weeks which may require a residential stay during the intensive follow-up period. For clinical trials involving patients receiving treatments already available in clinical care in phase 3 trials or equivalent, the closer the follow-up schedule is to routine clinical care, the easier it is to implement. For example, if patients typically are reviewed at the hospital 3 months after their treatment, then aligning the research visit and any associated additional testing and hospital-led data collection is more convenient for the participants than having to have a separate research visit on another day. It is important to make sure the collection of the primary outcome data is prioritized along with adequate procedures for collecting safety data.

Safety data collection and reporting

In addition to the specified outcomes which will typically include most or all anticipated harms which might affect a participant, a process for collecting any safety-related issues is needed. In the context of CTIMPS, this is called pharmacovigilance. Pharmacovigilance also continues in a different form for licensed IMPs outside of clinical trials. Beyond IMPs, collection of relevant safety data is still critical. It is important to note that relevant data are needed to be collected and assessed as a safety event irrespective of whether the event might be collected otherwise as an outcome. For example, all-cause mortality is a common outcome, particularly in oncology trials. Nevertheless, each death needs to be assessed as a safety event even though it may also be an outcome event (45). There is a clear difference in expectations and terminology regarding whether a trial is evaluating an IMP or not (i.e. the trial is a CTIMP or not). Most of the language used in discussing safety reporting and assessment are made with the presumption that an IMP or other drug-like product is being evaluated. A distinction is made between an adverse event and an adverse reaction: the latter is considered related to an IMP, the former may not be. The legal definition in the UK (and EU) in CTIMP legislation defines an 'adverse event' as 'any untoward medical occurrence in a subject to whom a medicinal product has been administered, including occurrences which are not necessarily caused by or related to that product' (3). Whereas an 'adverse reaction' is more narrowly defined as 'the means any untoward and unintended response in a subject to an investigational medicinal product which is related to any dose administered to that subject' (3). These definitions cover everything from the mildest to the most extreme, but possible, safety events. Each clinical trial therefore needs to be considered carefully in terms of the potential risk to participants. What is currently known about the treatments being evaluated, what is addressed within any related routine care, what can be expected, and how any unexpected event will be identified and escalated appropriately, need consideration. A process to log safety events at any point in the participants' involvement in the trial is needed.

Key pieces of information need to be collected for safety events. These include a description of what occurred and when, and whether the event is of an unexpected nature or not (e.g. some drug reactions will be anticipated but hoped to be rare or at least no more common than alternative drugs). Furthermore, the severity of the event, and whether it might be related to the trial treatments or the participants' more general involvement in the trial or not should be assessed. Any treatment received due to the event along with the final resolution should be recorded. Severity is assessed with regard to its impact and events which are fatal, life-threatening, lead to hospitalization or the prolongation of an existing hospitalization, result in persistent or significant disability or incapacity, or lead to congenital abnormality or birth defect are automatically considered 'severe' in the UK and the EU. Events which are thought to be related to the trial treatments or trial participation, as well as considered 'severe' are of most concern. This is particularly true for those which are 'unexpected' if it is also severe and potentially related to the study drug (potential 'causality' due to the IMP). In the UK and EU, these are called a 'suspected unexpected serious adverse response' (SUSAR), and in the US there are equivalent procedures to deal with this special type of adverse responses (3,45,46). 'Unexpected' would be considered in light of those events stated to be known adverse events in the investigator's brochure (or SmPC if the drug has marketing authorization), not that it is 'unlikely' or 'uncommon'. For trials of non-IMPs, a list of expected events would normally be listed in the protocol or in a related document and referenced accordingly to avoid considering any adverse event as one that needs to be reported on and addressed in an urgent manner.

An early phase trial will be anticipated to collect more information on adverse events reflecting that less will be known about the impact of the intervention(s) under evaluation. Sponsors will be responsible for taking action to address any unforeseen but immediate hazard to the health or safety of participants related to their participation. For a trial of an IMP, there will typically be strict timelines for reporting to the ethical review body, and the relevant regulatory approval body. For example, in the UK a life-threatening or SUSAR that results in a death must be reported to the MHRA with 7 days of the investigator being aware of it (47), or for other SUSAR events within 15 days (3). In order to meet such a timetable, sponsor and host institutions may have tighter reporting windows (e.g. 24 or 48 hours). For other types of clinical trials conducted in the UK, these will almost certainly require ethical review by the National Research Ethics Service. Accordingly, any serious adverse event which is considered to be potentially related to the study and unexpected would similarly be expected to be reported promptly (e.g. within 15 days). Aside from the reporting of some events of particular concern, it may be necessary to take urgent safety measures in order to protect study participants without prior authorization from a regulatory body though relevant bodies would be expected to be notified immediately of the change. In addition to the expedited reporting, there will be expectations regarding reporting of expected, and/or other non-life threatening, events of a serious nature. For example, the relevant ethical board may require annual reporting of progress including the occurrence of safety events (as RECs operating under the NHS's National Ethics Review Service do). CTIMPs with MHRA approval are required to complete an annual safety form (development safety update report) (47). The process for handing both expedited and regular safety reporting should be detailed in the protocol including how, and by whom, categorizations will be made, and how regularly they will be reported to relevant bodies.

Setting up research centres

Once the protocol is developed and overall regulatory approvals are in place (e.g. MHRA, ethics, and sponsor), the process of setting up research centres (or sites as they are sometimes called) can begin. Preliminary work of scoping out potential centres needs to begin early in the set-up process if not even earlier (e.g. as part of preparing a funding proposal) and not left until this point. Ultimately, it is only with the completeness of the set-up, the activation of recruitment at that centre, and indeed recruitment of participants from a centre, do we ultimately find out if the centre was a good choice or not. There are many problems and stumbling blocks in the way between a positive initial response from a centre declaring an interest in being involved, and a centre which is open for recruitment, let alone actively recruiting. The process, like other areas of clinical trials, has become increasingly bureaucratic over the last 20 years with little sign of that changing in the near future. This has been driven by an understandable concern for patient safety leading to a desire to ensure everything is in order prior to activating the centre. Another limiting step is the need for contracting and that each organization wants to ensure it is sufficiently protected. Specific documentation and processes will vary depending upon the clinical trial type (CTIMP, medical device, or other clinical trial), the sponsor's requirements, and the research centre's own processes.

Key tasks in setting up a new centre

- Appointment of a PI at the centre. One individual is usually required to be named who takes overall responsibility for the centre's involvement in the clinical trial. This individual will normally be a senior medical doctor with appropriate specialization (e.g. orthopaedic surgeon for a trial of knee surgery).
- Relevant approvals for the centre's participation have been agreed (e.g. an agreement between sponsor and centre detailing responsibilities). A study-specific confidentiality agreement may be requested.
- Collation of documentation to confirm suitability of the PI and other key centre staff (e.g. CV, medical certification/registration numbers). Evidence of specific insurance may also be required.
- Confirmation that any centre-specific materials (e.g. modified patient information sheets with different contact details, possibly different

information related to trial processes like advertisements) have appropriate approval.

- Specific responsibilities within the centre to complete relevant trial-related activities will need to be confirmed. While the PI will retain overall responsibility for the involvement of the centre in the clinical trial, specific tasks will usual be delegated or shared with a number of other staff members at each centre. For example, the process of introducing patients to the study, confirming patient eligibility, and overseeing consent and completion of care report forms may well be handled in part or fully by other members of staff (e.g. centre research coordinator appointed to the clinical trial) for at least some patients. Accordingly, a centre delegation log can be used to record the names, roles, and responsibilities of such individuals.
- Confirmation that all relevant materials (including the IMP) have been provided to the centre and are being stored appropriately.
- Providing a process of training relevant centre staff about the clinical trial objectives, relevant clinical trial processes (e.g. trial-specific operating processes related to administering the intervention), documentation (e.g. patient information leaflet for prospective participants, consent form, and centre completed and relevant participant completed forms), and systems (e.g. database) with which they will need to interact.

Making changes to the study once approved

It is common for some changes to be made to a clinical trial during its conduct. Key personnel may change, processes might need to be refined, or new processes may be introduced. The locations in which the trial is running may change with new centres initiated and others ceased. Alternatively, more fundamental changes to the scientific design might be needed due to new evidence from recently published studies. For example, a new outcome might be introduced, or less commonly the treatments under evaluation need some adjustment. Such changes, like the original protocol, require appropriate approvals as the original approvals are for the study to be conducted as submitted. For an IMP trial, any changes to the protocol or related documentation (e.g. care report form) will require notification to the MHRA (or FDA in the US for the equivalent type of trial) outlining what the changes are, clearly stating how wording has changed between versions, the reasons for the changes, and relevant supporting documentation (e.g. summaries of relevant data showing a problem such as missing data). The only exception to this, as noted earlier, is the implementation of urgent safety measures which can be implemented without prior approval though immediate notification of the relevant body is required. Perhaps less intuitively, stopping, suspending, or restarting a trial all also require notification to the relevant regulatory body, and in a similar manner the reasoning for doing so needs to be made clear. Finally, a declaration of the end of the study is required by relevant bodies. For CTIMPs and medical device clinical trials in the UK, both the MHRA and the REC will need to be notified of the end of the study. Other bodies may also need to be notified. As before, officially the sponsor is responsible for doing so but in practice the task is often delegated to other individuals. The sponsor will therefore need to be keep informed and engaged in the process of making any changes to the study.

Summary

Setting up a clinical trial is a daunting and increasingly complex task. In general, it is no longer the endeavour of a small number of investigators and instead requires a large team with a range of expertise. Having experience in study set-up and navigating regulatory approvals is key to keeping to schedule. Working with an experienced trials group (e.g. clinical trials unit in the UK or coordinating centre in the US) with a track record of delivery will ease the path for a new or relatively inexperienced clinical investigator seeking to lead their first clinical trial. Different types of clinical trials (phases, treatments, and study design) may require investigators and research support staff with fairly specific skills and expertise. A key step in the set-up is the process of converting a trial proposal into the finalized protocol. This requires care and attention to detail to address the scientific specifics of design, the practicalities of implementation, and also to ensure there is appropriate safeguarding of participants and their data.

References

1. Farrell B, Kenyon S, Shakur H. Managing clinical trials. Trials. 2010;11:78.
2. European Medicines Agency. Good clinical practice. 2021. Available from: https://www.ema.europa.eu/en/human-regulatory/research-development/compliance/good-clinical-practice
3. Legislation.gov.uk. The Medicines for Human Use (Clinical Trials) Regulations 2004. 2004. Available from: https://www.legislation.gov.uk/uksi/2004/1031/contents/made

4. Medicines and Healthcare products Regulatory Agency. Clinical trials for medicines: apply for authorisation in the UK. 2021. Available from: https://www.gov.uk/guidance/clinical-trials-for-medicines-apply-for-authorisation-in-the-uk

5. Pfeiffer J, Wells C. A Practical Guide to Managing Clinical Trials. Boca Raton, FL: CRC Press; 2020.

6. Holbein MEB. Understanding FDA regulatory requirements for investigational new drug applications for sponsor-investigators. Journal of Investigative Medicine. 2009;57(6):688–94.

7. European Medicines Agency. Clinical trials in human medicines. 2021. Available from: https://www.ema.europa.eu/en/human-regulatory/research-development/clinical-trials-human-medicines

8. European Medicines Agency. EU clinical trials register 2021. Available from: https://www.clinicaltrialsregister.eu/

9. International Council for Harmonisation of Technical Requirements for Pharmaceuticals for Human Use. Homepage. 2023. Available from: https://www.ich.org/

10. Beard DJ, Davies LJ, Cook JA, MacLennan G, Price A, Kent S, et al. Total versus partial knee replacement in patients with medial compartment knee osteoarthritis: the TOPKAT RCT. Health Technology Assessment. 2020;24(20):1–98.

11. Medicines and Healthcare products Regulatory Agency. Notify the MHRA about a clinical investigation for a medical device. 2021. Available from: https://www.gov.uk/guidance/notify-mhra-about-a-clinical-investigation-for-a-medical-device

12. Food and Drug Administration. Investigational device exemption (IDE). 2021. Available from: https://www.fda.gov/medical-devices/how-study-and-market-your-device/investigational-device-exemption-ide

13. Health Research Authority. IRAS—Integrated Research Application System. 2021. Available from: https://www.myresearchproject.org.uk/

14. Information Commissioner's Office. Overview—data protection and the EU. 2021. Available from: https://ico.org.uk/for-organisations/dp-at-the-end-of-the-transition-period/overview-data-protection-and-the-eu/

15. Medicines and Healthcare products Regulatory Agency. Algorithm 1—is it a clinical trial of a medicinal product? 2021. Available from: https://assets.publishing.service.gov.uk/government/uploads/system/uploads/attachment_data/file/949145/Algorithm_Clean__1_.pdf.

16. Medicines and Healthcare products Regulatory Agency. The supply of unlicensed medicinal products ('specials'). MHRA Guidance Note 14. 2014. Available from: https://assets.publishing.service.gov.uk/government/uploads/system/uploads/attachment_data/file/373505/The_supply_of_unlicensed_medicinal_products__specials_.pdf

17. International Council for Harmonisation of Technical Requirements for Pharmaceuticals for Human Use (ICH). Efficacy guidelines. Available from: https://www.ich.org/page/efficacy-guidelines

18. International Organization for Standardization. ISO 14155:2020. Clinical investigation of medical devices for human subjects—good clinical practice. 2020. Available from: https://www.iso.org/iso-13485-medical-devices.html

19. NHS Health Research Authority. Use of human tissue in research. 2001. Available from: https://www.hra.nhs.uk/planning-and-improving-research/policies-standards-legislation/use-tissue-research/

20. NHS Health Research Authority. Gene therapy advisory committee. 2021. Available from: https://www.hra.nhs.uk/about-us/committees-and-services/res-and-recs/gene-therapy-advisory-committee/

21. Administration of Radioactive Substances Advisory Committee. About us. 2021. Available from: https://www.gov.uk/government/organisations/administration-of-radioactive-substances-advisory-committee/about

22. NHS Health Research Authority. Consent and participant information guidance. 2021. Available from: http://www.hra-decisiontools.org.uk/consent/principles-children.html
23. Food and Drug Administration. Code of Federal Regulations. Title 21, Chapter I, Part 56: Institutional Review Boards, Subpart A, General Provisions. 2021. Available from: https://www.ecfr.gov/current/title-21/chapter-I/subchapter-A/part-56
24. Wikipedia. Common Rule. 2021. Available from: https://en.wikipedia.org/wiki/Comm on_Rule
25. Food and Drug Administration. Code of Federal Regulations. Title 21, Chapter I, Subchapter A. 2021. Available from: https://www.ecfr.gov/current/title-21/chapter-I/sub chapter-A
26. MODEPHARMA. About investigational medicinal product dossiers. 2021. Available from: https://www.imp-dossier.eu
27. Datapharm. What is an SmPC: Datapharm. 2017. Available from: https://emcsupport.me-dicines.org.uk/support/solutions/articles/7000007888-what-is-an-smpc-
28. Philpott C, le Conte S, Beard D, Cook J, Sones W, Morris S, et al. Clarithromycin and endoscopic sinus surgery for adults with chronic rhinosinusitis with and without nasal polyps: study protocol for the MACRO randomised controlled trial. Trials. 2019;20(1):246.
29. SPIRIT Group. Guidance for clinical trials protocols: SPIRIT. 2021 Available from: https://www.spirit-statement.org/
30. International Stroke Trial Collaborative Group. The International Stroke Trial (IST): a randomised trial of aspirin, subcutaneous heparin, both, or neither among 19435 patients with acute ischaemic stroke. Lancet. 1997;349(9065):1569–81.
31. NHS. Does grapefruit affect my medicine? 2021. Available from: https://www.nhs.uk/com mon-health-questions/medicines/does-grapefruit-affect-my-medicine/.
32. Food and Drug Administration. Grapefruit juice and some drugs don't mix. 2021. Available from: https://www.fda.gov/consumers/consumer-updates/grapefruit-juice-and-some-drugs-dont-mix
33. Boutron I, Guittet L, Estellat C, Moher D, Hróbjartsson A, Ravaud P. Reporting methods of blinding in randomized trials assessing nonpharmacological treatments. PLoS Medicine. 2007;4(2):e61.
34. European Coronary Surgery Study Group. Coronary-artery bypass surgery in stable angina pectoris: survival at two years. Lancet. 1979;1(8122):889–93.
35. McCulloch P, Altman DG, Campbell WB, Flum DR, Glasziou P, Marshall JC, et al. No surgical innovation without evaluation: the IDEAL recommendations. Lancet. 2009;374(9695):1105–12.
36. Blencowe NS, Mills N, Cook JA, Donovan JL, Rogers CA, Whiting P, et al. Standardizing and monitoring the delivery of surgical interventions in randomized clinical trials. British Journal of Surgery. 2016;103(10):1377–84.
37. Craig P, Dieppe P, Macintyre S, Michie S, Nazareth I, Petticrew M. Developing and evaluating complex interventions: the new Medical Research Council guidance. BMJ. 2008;337:a1655.
38. Hoffmann TC, Glasziou PP, Boutron I, Milne R, Perera R, Moher D, et al. Better reporting of interventions: template for intervention description and replication (TIDieR) checklist and guide. BMJ. 2014;348:g1687.
39. Beard D, Price A, Cook J, Fitzpatrick R, Carr A, Campbell M, et al. Total or Partial Knee Arthroplasty Trial—TOPKAT: study protocol for a randomised controlled trial. Trials. 2013;14:292.
40. Dawson J, Fitzpatrick R, Murray D, Carr A. Questionnaire on the perceptions of patients about total knee replacement. Journal of Bone and Joint Surgery. British Volume. 1998;80(1):63–9.

41. COSMIN (COnsensus-based Standards for the selection of health Measurement INstrument). Homepage. 2021. Available from: https://www.cosmin.nl/

42. Whitham D, Turzanski J, Bradshaw L, Clarke M, Culliford L, Duley L, et al. Development of a standardised set of metrics for monitoring site performance in multicentre randomised trials: a Delphi study. Trials. 2018;19(1):557.

43. Insall JN, Dorr LD, Scott RD, Scott WN. Rationale of the Knee Society clinical rating system. Clinical Orthopaedics and Related Research. 1989;248:13–4.

44. EuroQol Research Foundation. Homepage. 2021. Available from: https://euroqol.org/

45. US Department of Health and Human Services, Food and Drug Administration. Safety reporting requirements for INDs and BA/BE studies. 2012. Available from: https://www.fda.gov/files/drugs/published/Safety-Reporting-Requirements-for-INDs-%28Investigational-New-Drug-Applications%29-and-BA-BE-%28Bioavailability-Bioequivalence%29-Studies.pdf

46. European Commission. Communication from the Commission—detailed guidance on the collection, verification and presentation of adverse event/reaction reports arising from clinical trials on medicinal products for human use ('CT-3') 2011/C 172/01. Document 52011XC0611(01). 2011. Available from: https://eur-lex.europa.eu/LexUriServ/LexUriServ.do?uri=OJ:C:2011:172:0001:0013:EN:PDF

47. Medicines and Healthcare products Regulatory Agency. Clinical trials for medicines: manage your authorisation, report safety issues. 2021. Available from: https://www.gov.uk/guidance/clinical-trials-for-medicines-manage-your-authorisation-report-safety-issues

7

Data collection and monitoring in a clinical trial

> Statistical analysis of poor data is tantamount to attempting to make a silk purse out of a sow's ear.
>
> **Walter Modell and Raymond Houde, 1958 (1,2)**

Data, data, and more data

In Chapter 6 we considered the process of setting up a clinical trial including seeking the appropriate approvals needed to conduct the study. Here we return to the process of data collection, and ensuring all the data needed for the clinical trial (whether for monitoring, analysis, reporting, or interpretation) are being gathered. Along with the protocol, a substantial number of different forms (whether electronic or paper) will be needed to gather the relevant information required for the clinical trial. Furthermore, a database in which the trial data will be stored will also be needed. Before getting into the detail it is worth emphasizing that a clinical trial can only be as good as its data. It does not matter how well designed it is if the data are not available, appropriate, and of sufficient quality—it is to no avail. Data collection and monitoring is a critical stage in delivering a clinical trial; the approach should be tailored to reflect the objectives of the clinical trial. The overarching aim should be to ensure as far as possible the critical data are collected, missing data are minimized, and the data collected are accurate. We now consider in turn the different potential sources from which data may be collected, setting up the database we will need to store the data, how to plan to minimize missing data, and data monitoring, including interim analyses of data.

Data collection

Data sources

Data can be received from a variety of sources though typically most data comes from study-specific forms called case report forms (CRFs) which collect data on the participants. Other relevant sources of data include patient medical records, laboratory test reports, and imaging scans or other outputs of medical devices and tests. Participant blood samples may be taken on site but then sent to a laboratory for analysis. Alternatively, an imaging scan may be carried out at the trial centre (e.g. X-ray) but the output is sent for central review to ensure appropriate and standardized assessment. It is also common for key, more subjective assessments of clinical events (e.g. cardiovascular event) to be performed initially at the trial centre but for the assessment to be 'verified' or 'adjudicated' by a central review process. Each of the different processes will need to be addressed appropriately so that the required data are available for auditing, analysis, and reporting purposes. Unlike most clinical data which will be handled individually for each participant, data from such sources may well be dealt with in batches. The frequency and the nature of any corresponding data transfers need to be agreed in advance. Irrespective of where the data comes from, a key decision to be made is the degree to which the original information is collected and stored centrally at the trial office. See Chapter 8 for consideration of the administration of clinical trials including maintaining the trial master file (TMF). Commonly, the key data of interest are extracted from data sources by appropriately trained individuals, recorded onto a CRF (typically a paper one), and then later entered into the trial database.

One of the unfulfilled hopes in academic clinical trials over the last 10 years or so has been the utilization of routine data sources for clinical trial outcome follow-up. In one sense, use of 'routinely collected data' is not new as from early on clinical trials have made use of medical records to collect data related to patients. The main distinction is that these would then be reviewed to extract the data of interest, which was then transferred on to a trial CRF, or more recently entered directly into the trial database. Healthcare institutions are increasingly using electronic system to record not only diagnoses and use of treatments but also to a lesser extent health system quality measures and clinical outcomes. The ability to link trial participants to this data source so that the data do not need to be collected afresh for the clinical trial is attractive from a cost- and time-efficiency perspective. However, to date there has been limited use in clinical trials, and it is not used in trials intended to be part of a regulatory submission due to the difficulties in providing a full audit record, and to be able to fully ensure data quality. Furthermore, systems have tended to work in insolation making it difficult to implement across multiple sites. In the UK, there are routine data collection systems for England, Wales, and Scotland which record hospital and outpatient usage (3–5). An increasing number of primary care (family doctor) practices contribute data to a large database called the Clinical Practice Research Datalink (CPRD) with data on over 15 million patients (6). Death data are available UK wide from the Office of National Statistics, and other specialist databases often link to it to incorporate these data on the relevant people (6). While containing data on a very large numbers of individuals, the data are relatively shallow for most clinical conditions, and outcome data are very limited. Clinical registries (such as the National Hip Fracture Database in the UK) can be a richer source of data on the relevant clinical populations for clinical trials (7). This very much varies according to the clinical area, and the specific research question of interest (e.g. only limited short-term outcomes are often available). Patient-reported and quality of life outcomes tend to rarely be routinely collected and where they are, they are often not to a sufficient standard to be useful (e.g. low responses rates of 50% or less). There are some exceptions, and a number of the COVID-19 trials have made greater use of routine data from healthcare systems and relevant clinical registries (e.g. RECOVERY in the UK (8)) though this reflects the key outcomes focused on (e.g. mortality and hospitalization).

Determining what study data collection tools are needed

There is a fairly standard set of forms which are tailored to a specific trial to collect data related to specific trial events. These are the consent form, withdrawal form, adverse event form, and death notification form. In addition, there will be a number of forms for collecting key data at the specific time point of interests for participants. Sometimes the same form can be used for multiple time points, but mostly (even though much of the information is similar to another form) a specific form is needed due to the additional collection of further data points, and differences in the time gap between the points of data collection. Finally, there will sometimes be one-off disease or treatment event-related forms that may be required. For example, in a surgical trial, specific details related to any further operations might be collected on a specific form which is only completed for patients who go on to have a further operation. Alternatively, patients who have a flare-up in their condition (e.g. asthma) might be requested to complete a form related to it. Both of these forms relate to events that may or may not happen to a participant, and if they do, it will be at different points in the follow-up. Therefore, the process of dealing with such forms has to be different from that for the routine CRFs.

A key step in the process is thinking through the different pathways that patients could go through and ensuring that no key events or vital pieces of information will be missed if the planned processes are followed. For the initial approach and assessment of eligibility we need to ask how patients are to be identified, is any pre-screening assessment needed, and once screened, when and how is eligibility to be confirmed? Furthermore, we want to know how the consent process will be implemented, how consent will be recorded, and what information should be collected at the time of consent for those who have agreed to take part. Once an individual has consented to be in the study, how will their baseline data be collected, how will data on the treatment received be collected, and when and how are outcomes to be assessed? All of these questions need a clear answer. All data that needs to be collected have to have an associated paper form or another trial data source on which it is recorded (e.g. it could be directly entered into the trial database immediately after a measurement is taken). The protocol and associated trial-specific guidance accordingly needs to clarify which study forms are needed, who will complete then, and when they are to be completed.

Creating the case report forms and other trial data collection tools

Once the list of CRFs and other trial forms (e.g. screening and consent) and data entry tools have been confirmed, each form will need to be created. Care and attention are needed to make the form as self-explanatory as possible, and quick and easy to complete. Deciding what data can reasonably be collected on the same CRF with regard to length of form, the availability of information to complete at the same point in the participant's journey in the study, and who will complete the form are also key considerations. This process of generating the CRFs may well identify problems with the planned approach and may lead to some changes in which form specific data are collected on. It could lead to the creation of new forms to produce a smooth and complete data collection process.

All drafted CRFs and other forms need to undergo a review process before they are sent for formal ethical review and use in a clinical trial. The level of understanding that can be taken for granted will vary depending upon who is completing the form. Any participant-completed form needs particular care in generation to avoid the unnecessary use of jargon, or to collect data in a way that may exclude patients who have less knowledge about their condition. Having the form read through by someone external to the trial team is particularly helpful. Any 'patient-facing' forms would benefit from being reviewed by patients with the same or a similar condition, or other members of the public. The ideal form is one that can be completed by one individual in a single sitting in the intuitive order, that is, front to back on a paper form, or top to bottom if completed electronically. The need to backtrack or check other sections of the form should be avoided as far as possible. A form that needs to be returned to alter as some data cannot be completed the first time is more likely to be returned late, partially completed, or not completed at all. Where more than one individual's input is required (e.g. there is a pathologist's section as well as a research nurse's), distinct sections that are clearly labelled are needed to make it obvious for the relevant individuals what they should complete. If substantial input is needed from two or more individuals, separate forms might be the better option.

As with many things in life, the art of producing CRFs lies in finding a balance between collecting all the key information needed for the trial while resisting the urge to collect other, interesting information, that is not strictly needed. Overall, less is often more, as less to be collected makes correct completion of the form more likely, and it also makes the process of producing the CRF, setting up and testing the database, and cleaning the corresponding data quicker. As the process of setting up clinical trials has become more process driven, the impact of additional data adds up. Increasingly, electronic data collection is being used in clinical trials, that is, an electronic CRF (eCRF), as opposed to a hard copy (paper) CRF. While the digital revolution has changed many things greatly, and in many ways for the better, the shift to electronic data collection in clinical trials has been much slower and less successful than many initially anticipated. Getting something that works for everyone has been difficult (e.g. working and appearing well on a smart phone, tablet, as well as desktop computers). Making the most of the advantages of electronic data collection can be more time-consuming when setting up the system (e.g. automatic data range checks, hiding questions, and skipping sections based upon previous responses). The same general considerations in CRF development apply to electronic forms though checks of accessibility and testing need to be adapted to the format. We will consider this further as we think about setting the clinical trial database.

Setting up the clinical trial database

Typically, clinical trials will have their own database set-up specifically for the clinical trial. While many aspects may be common between trials, clinical trials are unique projects and vary in subtle ways regarding the data required and the processes to be followed. How the data will be stored needs to be considered early in the set-up process. A range of systems can be used to collect, manage, analyse, and report clinical trial data ranging from using basic spreadsheet (e.g. Microsoft Excel) through to comprehensive and bespoke databases (e.g. set-up using REDCaP, OpenClinica, or Oracle platform). The choice will depend upon the specific trial and the financial and host institution resources available. Increasingly, more in-depth processes of recording changes to the data are required for auditing purposes. Clinical trials that are conducted with a view to producing evidence for a regulatory approval application (such as a CTIMP evaluating an IMP without marketing approval) need to meet particularly high requirements for data verification and auditing by regulators. Therefore a database system that logs exactly when changes are made, by whom, and what the changes were is needed. This provides a clear audit trial available to be viewed by those who may be interested. Given the amount of data being collected some changes to the data are inevitable. Human error when entering data may be identified later through an audit review as the value may be obviously out of range, or be impossible via cross-checking with related data. For example, incompatible dates might be identified where an IMP was supposedly being received before the patient entered the study due to mis-entry of the date.

The advantages of electronic data collection are obvious: no need for an intermediary, and any potential misunderstanding, and no human error from subsequent data entry. Data systems can have checks implemented to ensure critical fields are completed, or values fall within credible ranges (e.g. follow-up data collection dates are post baseline). Some fields which are only relevant based upon a previous answer can be automatically skipped. Each of these steps and rules needs to be stipulated. However, there has been a number of obstacles to its regular use, as accessibility of IT equipment (e.g. a charged tablet or laptop) as and when needed brings some practical challenges and potentially the need for trial-specific equipment. Ensuring data protection requires user login and security to avoid data breaches. The challenges of having a system that works on different IT set-ups (both operating systems and web browsers if accessed that way) adds further challenges. Alternatively, producing specific apps can be costly.

Increasing use of smartphones and access to the internet is both a blessing and a curse for data collection. In theory, data are more accessible than ever and participants are more readily contactable. However, making something easy to read on a variety of screen sizes (particularly smartphones) and to complete is much more difficult than it initially appears. For some pieces of information (e.g. taking consent) there has been hesitancy from ethics review bodies to move away from paper-based forms as they might be viewed as providing greater reassurance about the participant's full consent having been given. Nevertheless, electronic data collection has become more common for at least part of the data collection for clinical trials. In particular, using an electronic system to oversee randomization, along with data collected by centre staff entered electronically, is becoming the norm for larger clinical trials. For implementation of randomization in particular, an electronic system offers a number of benefits and protections over a paper-based system (e.g. use of opaque envelopes) as we considered in Chapter 3. An electronic system practically precludes the possibility of tampering with the sequence generation. It can ensure any randomization is automatically logged including when and by whom (at least what login was used). Any additional data required or which needs to verified can be requested prior to randomization. Furthermore, it could automatically implement more complex randomization methods (e.g. stratification through to minimization or outcome response-based approaches as covered in Chapter 3). Whatever randomization system is used, like the checks of any paper CRFs being used in the trial, the database will need to have undergone a thorough process of checking prior to use. More critical systems (e.g. randomization) will need more extensive testing prior to use.

Typically, the database will be structured to reflect the data entry forms and other data sources. In the past, annotated CRFs were often used to explicitly state the name of the relevant data field to which specific CRF question responses related to. Data matrices or dictionaries are now more commonly used as part of the database build to specify what each field should be called, how it should be defined, and what types of response are permitted. These should be maintained and updated to reflect changes made during the conduct of a clinical trial so that they are available to facilitate data sharing following the closure of the trial. Requested checks can be indicated along with any required calculations. For example, the date of birth can be requested and the exact format specified. The resultant age on the date of data entry can then be automatically calculated. An automatic check could also be made to ensure, for example, the entered age is, say, at least 18 years. As far as possible, each item of data should only be entered once unless it is an intentional check to ensure the correct value has been received. A well-designed system will anticipate where specific data are not applicable for some participants, and whether data should be available or not. For example, it may be necessary to confirm if a specific sample for a laboratory test was carried out or not, and if not, the relevant questions are not requested to be completed. Use of text boxes which allow text responses should be used sparingly, as text provided for participants can be irrelevant (to the specific question of interest), difficult to decipher (even when electronically completed), and they are more time-consuming to complete (clean and analyse). The response from text boxes will often need specialist review (e.g. senior medical doctor). The use of multiple-choice questions with appropriate options can limit such free text use to an 'other' category for which a text box is used to provide details.

Planning to minimize missing data

Some missing data are inevitable in even the best conducted clinical trials. However, those which are well designed and conducted will minimize such occurrences. Missing data are a threat to the scientific integrity of the trial, either by undermining the statistical analysis or by generating uncertainty in the interpretation of the findings. For example, if some of the key baseline data points are missing, such as age and key comorbidities, it can obscure who the results pertain to and make clinical application problematic. Missing data in general will reduce the statistical precision of any analysis, though to an extent this can be compensated for (though with a corresponding increase in work-load). Of particular concern is the introduction of any bias between groups, that is, the missing data mechanism (cause or pattern) differs between the in-tervention and control groups. In particular, any difference in the approach to data collection between the intervention and control groups needs to be carefully considered as it has the potential to influence participants' behaviour and responses. This then has an impact upon the summary results and potentially the findings of the study. An additional prompt to assess the inter-vention group may influence participants' compliance with the intervention treatment and could alter the participants' behaviour. Alternatively, routine clinical follow-up patterns that may be reasonable for clinical practice might not be suited to a clinical trial. They could implicitly collect more information on the intervention than the control or vice versa. For placebo-blinded clinical trials, and early phase clinical trials, this is less of a concern as the clinical trial is less directly relevant to clinical practice and less open to influence as a more strict, though artificial, schedule of clinical care is likely to be followed. The key to mitigating the potential impact of missing data is thinking through the trial data collection and identifying potential problematic aspects in advance.

There are at least three approaches which can play a part to mitigate missing data. First, the consent form and withdrawal (or perhaps better called a change of consent) forms should make a distinction between consent for treatment and consent for data collection. The latter can often be further usefully sep-arated out into active and passive data collection (e.g. available from medical staff at site without requiring the participant to attend a study visit, or to com-plete forms). The term 'withdrawal' can easily be misunderstood and be too readily interpreted as complete cessation of any further involvement in the clinical trial. Often a participant may for various reasons feel they do not want to continue to receive the trial treatment, receive further information on the study, or complete further forms. However, they may well still be content for the trial team to collect data from clinical sources which do not require their active involvement. Second, the way data collection tools are designed and delivered needs careful consideration to make complete and accurate completion as easy as possible. Training of centre staff can play a part in this and it can emphasize the importance of collecting specific data and the detrimental impact upon the trial's scientific credibility, and, where relevant, the impact upon patient safety. Third, data collection needs to prioritize the critical data over the desirable data. Allowing participants to provide only part of data desired can be beneficial. Correspondingly, chasing up only on the most important data following non-response to letters, emails, or texts, may be warranted to reduce the burden on the participants and study personnel. In particular, the value of continuing to collect data on participants who have stopped their treatment (where permission to do so has not been removed, i.e. the participant has not withdrawn consent to follow-up) needs to be communicated to study staff and participants. Similarly for participants who have missed a previous study visit or discontinued treatment, the value of continuing to collect data is not necessarily intuitive to many involved with clinical trials.

Data monitoring

Having considered the setting-up of the data collection system, consideration now turns to data monitoring, a critical aspect of clinical trial conduct in order to ensure the quality of data for analyses and reporting and to ensure patient safety. More formally, it can be described broadly as 'the act of overseeing the progress of a clinical trial, and of ensuring that is it conducted, recorded, and reported in accordance with the protocol, Standard Operating Procedures (SOPs), GCP, and the applicable regulatory requirement(s)' (9). Monitoring of data collection is just one area of monitoring of the conduct of a clinical trial that might be done.

Data audits

A similar though distinct activity to monitoring is auditing. The ICH guidelines define auditing as 'a systematic and independent examination of trial-related activities and documents to determine whether the evaluated trial-related activities were conducted, and the data recorded, analysed, and accurately reported accordingly to the protocol, sponsor's standard operation procedures (SOPs), GCP and the applicable regulatory requirement(s)' (9). Auditing may be done by the group running the trial (whether focused solely on a single trial or an aspect of trial conduct across a number of other studies). It may also be done on behalf of the sponsor (but independently of the investigators and trial group running the trial), or by an external body (e.g. by regulatory body such as the MHRA in the UK or the FDA in the US who will conduct in-depth reviews of clinical trials). These external audits tend to be one-off assessments and although they may identify issues with the data, they tend to be more process focused. The scope and specifics of the audit will vary greatly depending upon who instigates it and for what purpose (e.g. whether it is a regular audit or one initiated in response to some stated concerns). Most audits focus on the trial office and lead trial centre though queries may be raised that request involvement of other centres.

Data monitoring strategy

There are two main aspects to the monitoring of clinical trial data. First, it must be ensured that the required data are being collected. Second, the quality of the collected data must be verified. Processes needs to be in place to check in particular on critical data. As well as making sure the system minimizes data absences and errors as far as possible, systematic checks of the data are vital to ensure the quality of trial data. Scheduled checks are often planned to precede any key decision-making events (e.g. a meeting of a trial committee). Modification to the study protocol and data collection tools (e.g. CRFs) may be needed to address problematic issues identified when conducting checks. Alternatively, it may highlight the need for further training of centre staff in a particular part of the trial procedures and the use of certain forms. In addition to ensuring the trial data are of a high quality, monitoring also plays a key part in ensuring patient safety and identifying threats to the scientific integrity of the study. Inconsistencies in data may be identified which need to be queried with centres and they can be of clinical relevance to the participants' ongoing and future medical care. The extent and regularity of checks needs to be considered in light of the regularity of the use of the data and the potential consequences of errors. For example, in a clinical trial with a dose-escalation design, the presence of a toxicity event can lead to the stopping of the trial, or the changing of the dose for the next participant. Therefore, safety data in such a clinical trial require more regular checks to ensure each decision made is appropriate as the study proceeds. A further aspect to consider is the dual interest of data collected regarding a clinical event for a safety purpose, and also as it relates to an outcome to be included for the statistical analysis. For trials of some conditions (e.g. trials of treatment for cardiovascular disease where the typical clinical events of most interest are death, myocardial faction, stroke, hospitalization due to heart failure, etc.) there is substantial overlap between safety events and key outcomes of interest (e.g. primary outcome which might be time to the occurrence of the first MACE). However, for other conditions this is much less true and safety events concern treatment side effects (e.g. headache or fatigue). Interest in the event experienced as an outcome may be better collected by assessing the impact upon quality of life as opposed to the pure count and categorizations that are required for regulatory safety monitoring. Reviews of data can be conducted and/or overseen by the administrative lead for the study (e.g. trial manager or coordinator), by a trial management or coordination group, or by independent assessment (e.g. summary presented to an oversight or data safety and monitoring committee (see below for further consideration of this)). The trial statistician may also conduct reviews associated with key time points (e.g. preparing reports for a trial committee). A healthy data monitoring strategy will involve regular assessments at different levels of oversights. The strategy needs to take account of what is already known about the intervention and the control treatments, and the type of trial being conducted. For example, a phase 1 first-in-human trial with healthy volunteers clearly will need complete assessment of adverse events very regularly. In contrast, a phase 3 trial of an IMP which is already used for another indication can utilize substantial existing data on its safety profile to focus on safety data collection, while still allowing for the possibility of a SUSAR and monitoring of other serious adverse events. Furthermore, if the trial population has a chronic condition like type 1 diabetes, certain adverse events can be anticipated without raising undue concern (e.g. hypoglycaemia). Table 7.1 gives some examples of checks and problems that might be detected at different levels of review. Misunderstanding regarding aspects of the trial processes, and with regard to completion of forms, are common occurrences even with careful development of the data collection tools and training of centre staff. It is a very rare occurrence for scientific misconduct to be identified; nevertheless, checks of data can also identify issues with the patient consent process, or even if falsified data have been entered. In addition to seeking to 'reclaim' data whenever possible, data monitoring and associated checks may also lead to changes being implemented which will prevent, or attenuate, further occurrences of the same problem.

Table 7.1 Data monitoring schedule assessments

Level of assessment	Checks	Example problems that might be identified	Remedy
Trial manager/coordinator	Routine checks	Common absence of completion of a key data value when checking on patient status Data for a particular patient which is incompatible	Query with centre Correction of data entry where necessary
Regular trial administration meetings	Log of protocol deviations	Centre which is incorrectly applying trial processes	Query with centre to understand circumstances Further training may be appropriate
Trial Management Group (see Chapter 8)	Regular report of trial progress	Centre with a particular low return rate of a form compared to other centres	Query with centre to understand practices Further training may be appropriate
Trial Steering Committee (see Chapter 8)	Regular report of trial progress	Form returned much less commonly than in other trials with similar data collection methods	Identify any trial-specific aspect which could contribute Modify trial processes as appropriate Protocol amendment to implement a revised form to facilitate better completion
Data and Safety Monitoring Committee	Review of (closed) Data and Safety Monitoring Committee report	Problem with randomization indicated by imbalance between randomized groups	Isolate source of problem (data entry or randomization algorithm) Update randomization system as appropriate

Tracking data completion

A system for tracking a participant's data through their involvement in the clinical trial is a helpful tool in ensuring data quality. It will help with early identification of missing forms and data for particular patients. In addition, it will help to coordinate centre and trial staff. While such a process can be managed from use of a detailed spreadsheet, this is an area where a well-designed database can facilitate and substantially reduce the administrative burden on staff. For example, automatic reports may be readily produced which summarize the completion of key forms and potentially for critical data points within forms. Email and/or text message reminders could be automated to prompt in advance the respective individual (whether a participant or centre or trial staff member) to complete a specific task or to return a form, or as a reminder when they are overdue to allow it to be addressed in a timely manner.

Data monitoring schedule

An example data monitoring schedule is given in Table 7.2 for the Vaccine Response On/Off Methotrexate (VROOM) trial which sought to assess the impact of a 2-week suspension of taking an immunosuppressive drug (methotrexate) for patients who received a further 'booster' COVID-19 vaccine injection (10,11). As the study was anticipated to recruit quickly (within 12 months), the initial expectation was that the Data Safety and Monitoring Committee (DSMC) and Trial Steering Committee (TSC) would only meet a small number of times in the course of the trial. A Trial Management Group (TMG) involving only the core trial team was expected to meet monthly to review progress including recruitment and data collection. See later in the chapter for a discussion of the role of the DSMC, and in Chapter 8 for discussion of the TMG and the TSC. Some of the regular checks carried out by the relevant groups are shown in Table 7.2.

Interim analysis

An interim analysis is a formal statistical analysis which evaluates the safety and/or efficacy of the treatments under evaluation based upon the accumulated data part way through the study's conduct. A trial may have any number of interim analyses (including none) though generally the number of analyses is small in order for each to be more meaningful. It is important to distinguish between an interim analysis, in the sense that a statistical analysis will be carried out with a formal assessment of some form (e.g. carrying out a formal statistical analysis and seeking a specific, and stricter, i.e. lower, significance level in order to decide whether to recommend stopping or not), and any informal

Table 7.2 Data monitoring schedule example—VROOM trial

Responsible group	Check to be carried out	Frequency
Trial office	Various regular checks including:	
	• Patient registered interest and baseline visit not yet completed	Weekly
	• Missing/out-of-window follow-up case report forms	Weekly
	• Automated reminder to participants to provide key date by SMS upon which follow-up is dependent.	Weekly
	• Serious adverse events data	Immediate
	• Blood samples collected and sent to laboratory for processing	Periodically
Trial Management Group	Review of report on study progress including recruitment, and data collection information	Monthly during study set-up, recruitment, and follow-up
Data and Safety Monitoring Committee	Overview review of data quality and integrity. Interim analysis using Haybittle–Peto stopping guideline at a single time point once primary outcome 28-day data is available for 250 participants	Meet prior to study initiation and two times during the trial. Meeting timed to allow timely review of interim analysis. Received update summaries periodically in between
Trial Steering Committee	Review report on study progress, trial conduct, and safety data issues arising	Meet prior to study initiation and twice per year
Ethics committee	Summaries of serious adverse events Unexpected related serious adverse events	Annual Immediately reporting

assessment of accumulating data. While interim analyses may be carried out for a number of reasons, the most common are as follows:

1. To potentially stop the trial early if a conclusion can be reached regarding the primary objective of the study (e.g. the efficacy of the intervention treatment has clearly been shown in the statistical analysis).
2. To confirm progression to the next stage of the clinical trial according to its design (e.g. to determine the dose level for use in subsequent patients in a dose escalation study).
3. To provide a formal point at which the safety of the intervention treatment will be assessed.

Whether a clinical trial is to have any interim analysis should be clearly stated in the protocol. If it is, an outline of the approach should be stated. The responsibility for determining the finding of the interim analysis (e.g. a subset of the trial team, or external individuals), and who will make the decision based upon this should be stated in the trial documentation when the trial is set up. The statistical analysis plan (see Chapter 9) for a clinical trial should clearly address whether there will be any interim analysis, and, if so, of what nature. For more complex interim analyses, it may be useful to have a separate interim analysis statistical plan to fully cover all the relevant details and information for the interim analysis and related decision.

Many clinical trials will have a specific data committee. This DSMC will have responsibility for reviewing reports of accumulating data, the interpretation of any interim analyses, and making recommendations regarding the continuation and potential modifications to the trial (e.g. changing the inclusion criteria based upon findings or addressing inadequacies in the data) (13). Very similar names are used for the group that performs these functions (e.g. Data Monitoring Committee, Data Monitoring and Ethics Board). It is preferable that those who sit on such a committee and make recommendations where scientific merit and patient safety both have to be considered, are 'independent' to the trial investigators, that is, the committee does not include trial investigators and are without any direct ties institutional or otherwise to them. This is helpful if for no other reason than to avoid the perception of bias. Having a clear charter, detailing the way in which the committee will operate, is important in the event that decisions become contentious (14). A list of the potential specific roles the DSMC may take on prepared by the DAMOCLES group is given in Table 7.3 (12). Sponsors and regulatory bodies may have guidance about when and how they except such a committee to operate (15). The membership should include expertise in the intervention and control treatments, clinical trial conduct, and the monitoring of trial data.

For many phase 3 clinical trials, no interim analysis is carried out (though informal data monitoring will still occur, and may still be reviewed by a DSMC). This is often due to the timescale of the outcomes of interest being collected, the anticipated recruitment rate, and the overall sample size of their trial. Together they may mean there is no realistic likelihood of an interim analysis being useful. In contrast, some clinical trials are designed with the possibility of a substantial change in design part way through in mind (i.e. adaptive trials, as introduced in Chapter 4). Accordingly, they are often purposely designed with a pre-specified interim analysis in order to determine when and how the trial design should adapt given the accumulated data. Either way there is the potential for events to overtake the best laid designs, leading to a trial stopping early due to unforeseen concerns (e.g. the otherwise effective IMP seems to be causing strokes).

Table 7.3 List of roles for the Data Safety and Monitoring Committee

Overall role	Specific roles
Interim review of the trial's progress including updated figures on recruitment, data quality, and main outcomes and safety data	A selection of specific aspects could be compiled from the following list: • Assess data quality, including completeness (and by so doing encourage collection of high-quality data) • Monitor recruitment figures and losses to follow-up • Monitor compliance with the protocol by participants and investigators • Monitor organisation and implementation of trial protocol (the DSMC[a] should only perform this role in the absence of other trial oversight committees) • Monitor evidence for treatment differences in the main efficacy outcome measures • Monitor evidence for treatment harm (e.g. toxicity data, serious adverse events, deaths) • Decide whether to recommend that the trial continues to recruit participants or whether recruitment should be terminated, either for everyone or for some treatment groups and/or some participant subgroups • Suggest additional data analyses • Advise on protocol modifications suggested by investigators or sponsors (e.g. to inclusion criteria, trial end points, or sample size) • Monitor planned sample size assumptions • Monitor continuing appropriateness of patient information • Monitor compliance with previous DSMC recommendations • Consider the ethical implications of any recommendations made by the DSMC • Assess the impact and relevance of external evidence

DSMC, Data Safety and Monitoring Committee.

[a] Note—the original version used 'DMC' instead of DSMC.

Earlier in Chapters 3 and 5 it was noted that any statistical analysis runs the risk of producing a potentially misleading finding. With regard to stopping early, this is usually in regard to falsely concluding there is a benefit to the intervention treatment based upon the data available part way through the study. The more interim analyses that are carried out, the greater the risk of stopping early in error. To combat this, the statistical criteria applied to an interim analysis that could lead to stopping a trial early need to be stricter than those applied to the final analysis of the data. For example, a very strict two-sided significance level of 0.1% is commonly used (the Haybittle–Peto boundary) (10,11,16). This approach seeks to reflect the view that trials should only be stopped for a treatment difference if the statistical evidence is 'beyond reasonable doubt' as only then will it be likely accepted as a valid result, and could have the potential to influence clinical practice. Such criteria for stopping a clinical trial early have often been described as 'stopping rules', though more accurately they can be referred to as 'stopping guidelines'. No statistical analysis-based criteria are able to fully capture all relevant considerations related to stopping early or continuing a clinical trial. This must include wider considerations of patient safety and potential scientific value of the clinical trial continuing, and the influence of external evidence (which could go either way). Aside from these considerations, phase 3 clinical trials are designed to provide a clear answer ('confirmatory' or 'definitive'), and therefore should be designed to be in favour of continuing except where a compelling case for stopping can be made. Clinical trials that are intended for regulatory submissions are less likely to be compelling to a regulator if stopped early. Additionally, stopping clinical trials on the basis of only one outcome, even if it is the primary outcome, could prevent the full collection of sufficient data to address all the study objectives. Even from purely a scientific perspective, the decision to stop is therefore more complex than it might initially appear. Ethical considerations need to be weighed up according to the specifics of the clinical trial being conducted and what else is known, along with practical considerations of stopping a trial early.

Summary

Data monitoring is a key part of conducting a clinical trial and is critical for ethical, practical, and scientific reasons. Trial data quality cannot be taken for granted. A proactive approach is needed to ensure the completeness, validity, and reliability of collected trial data. The degree of monitoring required particularly regarding safety will vary greatly depending upon the type of trial, the phase of trial, what is already know about the intervention and control, and the trial design. An interim (statistical) analysis may play a useful part in the monitoring strategy, and any decision whether, and how, to continue a clinical trial or not part way through. As with other aspects of clinical trials, data monitoring should be planned in advance and reviewed periodically to ensure the study is conducted appropriately.

References

1. Modell W, Houde RW. Factors influencing clinical evaluation of drugs; with special reference to the double-blind technique. Journal of the American Medical Association. 1958;167(18):2190–9.

2. Cromie BW. The feet of clay of the double-blind trial. Lancet. 1963;2(7315):994–7.

3. NHS Digital. Hospital episode statistics. 2021. Available from: https://digital.nhs.uk/data-and-information/data-tools-and-services/data-services/hospital-episode-statistics

4. Public Health Scotland. Data and intelligence. 2020. Available from: https://www.isdscotland.org/

5. Health in Wales. Statistics and data. 2021. Available from: https://www.wales.nhs.uk/statisticsanddata

6. Clinical Practice Research Datalink. CPRD linked data. 2021. Available from: https://www.cprd.com/linked-data

7. Cook JA, Collins GS. The rise of big clinical databases. British Journal of Surgery. 2015;102(2):e93–101.

8. RECOVERY Collaborative Group. Dexamethasone in hospitalized patients with Covid-19. New England Journal of Medicine. 2021;384(8):693–704.

9. International Council for Harmonisation of Technical Requirements for Pharmaceuticals for Human use (ICH). Integrated addendum to ICH E6(R1): guideline for good clinical practice E6(R2). 2006. Available from: https://database.ich.org/sites/default/files/E6_R2_Addendum.pdf

10. Abhishek A, Boyton RJ, McKnight Á, Coates L, Bluett J, Barber VS, et al. Effects of temporarily suspending low-dose methotrexate treatment for 2 weeks after SARS-CoV-2 vaccine booster on vaccine response in immunosuppressed adults with inflammatory conditions: protocol for a multicentre randomised controlled trial and nested mechanistic substudy (Vaccine Response On/Off Methotrexate (VROOM) study). BMJ Open. 2022;12(5):e062599.

11. Abhishek A, Boyton RJ, Peckham N, McKnight Á, Coates LC, Bluett J, et al. Effect of a 2-week interruption in methotrexate treatment versus continued treatment on COVID-19 booster vaccine immunity in adults with inflammatory conditions (VROOM study): a randomised, open label, superiority trial. Lancet Respiratory Medicine. 2022;10(9):840–50.

12. Grant AM, Altman DG, Babiker AB, Campbell MK, Clemens FJ, Darbyshire JH, et al. Issues in data monitoring and interim analysis of trials. Health Technology Assessment. 2005;9(7):1–238, iii–iv.

13. Ellenberg SS, Fleming TR, DeMets DL. Data Monitoring Committees in Clinical Trials: A Practical Perspective. 2nd ed. Hoboken, NJ: Wiley; 2019.

14. DAMOCLES Study Group. A proposed charter for clinical trial data monitoring committees: helping them to do their job well. Lancet. 2005;365(9460):711–22.

15. Committee for Medicinal Products for Human Use (CHMP), European Medicines Agency. Guideline on data monitoring committees. 2005. Available from: https://www.ema.europa.eu/en/documents/scientific-guideline/guideline-data-monitoring-committees_en.pdf

16. Pocock SJ. When (not) to stop a clinical trial for benefit. JAMA. 2005;294(17):2228–30.

8

Conducting a clinical trial

> However well planned a clinical trial may be, it is useless unless the instructions are conscientiously and efficiently followed.
>
> **David Finney, 1964 (1)**

Now for the hardest part

Running a clinical trial is far from straightforward. It requires a myriad of decisions, actions, and tasks to be completed efficiently and quickly. This requires the input of a large number of people in various roles. In short, running a clinical trial is not for the faint-hearted. Furthermore, plenty of hard work, good management, and input from relevant experts are required to ensure its smooth running. Accordingly, in this chapter we will consider appropriate trial organization and oversight, how to get trial centres ready, maintaining trial documentation, dealing with protocol deviations and related events, along with the challenge of creating a successful recruitment and retention strategy.

Trial organization and oversight

Trials are complex and involve many different people often at different locations (even for a single-centre trial). As such, a single point of contact and administrative home for the clinical trial is essential to good conduct. Typically, an administrative centre, or 'trial office', is set up to serve this purpose. While the chief investigator will be to many the public face of the clinical trial, the practical contact will be the trial office. The office may in reality be predominantly one individual (e.g. trial manager or coordinator, or clinical researcher), or a small number of people through a system of support which provides cover as needed to maintain continuity. Very large trials and those intended for regulatory submission for approvals may have much larger teams due to the greater administrative and documentation burden involved.

Appropriate IT support is also critical to the successful running of a clinical trial, and will play a key role through the set-up and maintenance of the study database.

Different levels of oversight are needed to ensure appropriate and timely decision-making and action when conducting a clinical trial (2). While the sponsor is ultimately responsible for the conduct of the clinical trial (see Chapter 6 for further discussion of the role of the sponsor), these groups operate on behalf of the sponsor to ensure the clinical trial is conducted appropriately. Trial decision-making will typically operate at, at least, two levels. An oversight committee or TSC makes the 'big' strategic decisions (e.g. to stop the trial, change the eligibility criteria pending regulatory approvals, etc.). Additionally, there is a more regular TMG which deals with more mundane but pertinent issues related to the smooth running of the clinical trial. We will consider in turn these two core groups though we note they may well be supplemented by meetings with all the trial investigators, and operational subgroups of trial staff with/without the chief investigator, meeting on a regular or ad hoc basis as needed. As with all trial activities, careful documentation of decision-making is key to ensuring decisions are implemented appropriately.

A single oversight or coordinating committee will typically make the key decisions related to the conduct of the clinical trial (2). This body is usually called the TSC in UK NHS/charity-funded and academic-led studies. The TSC monitors trial progress and conduct, and provides advice on the scientific aspects of the study. Its membership should ideally include both members of the trial team (e.g. the chief investigator and some others) and external experts (e.g. experienced clinical researchers with substantial expertise in the treatments under evaluation and conducting clinical trials). A list of the specific roles the TSC may take on is given in Table 8.1 (3). Depending upon the sponsor of the study and the funding arrangement, there may be specific expectations about who will be involved in the committee (even down to the proportion of 'independent' members). Including patients or members of the public on this body is becoming more common in academic-led studies. It is also becoming more common for the membership to cover expertise in areas such as health economics and qualitative research in addition to the core areas of clinical knowledge, conduct of trials, and medical statistics. The TSC, or equivalent, is responsible for the oversight of the clinical trial from initiation to completion. The TMG and data and safety monitoring committee (the DSMC, if it exists) report to the TSC. They make recommendations regarding the conduct of the study for the TSC to consider (e.g. modifications to the trial protocol). In some trials, a separate DSMC is not necessary, and the TSC will take on some of the specific roles of a DSMC. The TSC needs to meet

Table 8.1 List of roles for the Trial Steering Committee

Overall role	Specific roles
To act as the oversight body for the trial on behalf of the sponsor and funder	• Provide expert oversight of the trial • Monitor the overall conduct of the trial, ensuring that it follows the standards set out in the guidelines of good clinical practice • Review and approve the protocol and other study documentation (e.g. case report forms and statistical analysis plan) • Review regular reports of the trial (prepared by the Trial Management Group) • Decide on the continuation of the trial • Monitor recruitment and retention levels • Review adherence to the protocol by investigators and participants • Receive and consider the recommendations of the Data Safety and Monitoring Committee • Assess the impact and relevance of external evidence • Monitor completeness of data • Review and approve substantive protocol amendments and any related proposals which change the design of the trial (e.g. an additional substudy) • Approve the main trial manuscript and key trial publications • Approve external or internal requests for release of data or subsets of data or samples *Additional responsibilities may include:* • Endorse the annual report to the funder and ethics (if required), and any related funding requests • Approve main presentation of trial results • Approve strategies to improve recruitment or retention

regularly enough to be able to review the trial's progress and make key decisions (e.g. the continuation or stopping of the study's recruitment, or moving to a new stage in the trial such as from phase 1 to phase 2) as well as contribute to the reporting of the findings. As with the DSMC as discussed in Chapter 7, a charter is useful for agreeing the terms of reference for the group and voting rights where formal decisions are needed. The frequency of meetings will vary from trial to trial though rates of once every 6 months or perhaps every 12 months for longer running phase 3 trials in a steady stage are common.

The TMG will meet regularly during the conduct of the trial and has a more 'hands-on' role in the study conduct and management. Monthly meetings will typically be the minimum frequency required with ad hoc meetings convened as needed. This is due to the potential nature of the issues that may arise (e.g. an urgent safety issue requiring prompt action) and also the range of issues that may occur (e.g. from IMP manufacturing issues to centre-specific problems) when conducting a clinical trial. A substantial number of people may attend such a meeting though typically these will be the chief investigator, trial administrative staff (e.g. trial manager or coordinator, data manager, and administrative support), and the trial statistician. Other individuals with trial expertise, or other investigators, may attend regularly, or as needed. This group will monitor the progress of the trial in terms of approvals, study set-up, recruitment, adherence to the trial protocol, safety issues, and any other relevant issue (e.g. initiation of another clinical trial recruiting from a similar patient population). Initial plans to address any issues identified would be the responsibility of this group along with preparing reports for the TSC, and where there is an issue of a significant nature, proposing a strategy to the TSC for approval.

Getting trial centres ready

Once all the appropriate approvals are in place, trial centres will need to be set up and staff trained in the specifics of the clinical trial. This includes familiarization of relevant staff in the study documentation and processes, and provision of relevant logins to the trial systems (e.g. randomization and database). Training of study centre staff in the processes of the trial will need to explore centre policies and practices to ensure it is clear what should be done and when at that specific centre. A particularly key aspect is ensuring centre staff are clear about safety monitoring requirements, and the need for clear and fast reporting of any safety event via the relevant CRF (e.g. serious adverse event). All supplies needed for the running of the trial (most importantly but not exclusively the IMP) will need to be shipped to a study centre. All of these actions need to occur for the centre to be 'activated', that is, to be in a position to start recruiting to the study. Supplies of the IMP along with other necessary items (e.g. blood sample collection kits) will need to be monitored by the trial office. This includes any relevant expiry dates, and supplies re-stocked as appropriate to avoid centres being unable to recruit due to lack of the IMP or consumables required for study participation. This may require additional manufacturing during the course of the trial to ensure the IMP is available in a timely manner when needed (whether due to expiry of the initial IMP or due to restocking given centre recruitment). The protocol and current versions of all trial documentation (e.g. patient information leaflet, consent form, and CRFs) need to be provided to centres in sufficient quantities, and replacements provided, and confirmation that superseded versions are disposed of, when they are updated.

Maintaining trial documentation

Expectation regarding the preparation, maintenance, and scope of trial documentation has substantially increased over the last 30 years. The TMF is the collection of all essential documents and records related to the conduct and management of the clinical trial. It should be sufficient to explain and provide all the trial data and show compliance with GCP and other relevant regulatory requirements (e.g. ethical approval). The UK legislation, which is based upon the corresponding ICH guideline, states 'all clinical trial information shall be recorded, handled, and stored in a way that allows its accurate reporting, interpretation and verification' (4,5). In the past there may have been a single physical 'file' kept in an appropriate location (e.g. trial office or pharmacy). The TMF for a modern clinical trial will now be part electronic and part physical. The TMF needs to be kept up to date and available for inspection (e.g. by host institution, sponsor, or regulatory bodies like the MHRA or FDA). It should be sufficient to allow reconstruction of the activities undertaken during the conduct of the trial and justification for actions taken. Clearly, the TMF will include the protocol, participant information leaflet, CRFs, and other trial forms (approved versions and potentially also completed forms). However, it also needs to encompass approval documentation, database information, analysis files, and trial output documents (e.g. trial reports and monitoring documentation). The TMF can then serve as an assurance and proof that the clinical trial has been conducted according to the principles of GCP. To ensure separation of data from investigators, statistical data, analysis files, and the database can be held separately and be accessible only to the relevant staff members while the trial is running. All the information sources are combined once the trial is complete. Trial centres will be similarly required to maintain their own centre files with relevant documentation (some of which will be duplicated with the TMF, and others may be solely kept at the study centre). A key step in the setting up of study centres is confirming what information has to be stored locally and what needs to be sent to the trial office for inclusion in the TMF.

Protocol deviations, violations, and serious breaches

The protocol as approved by the ethics committee and other regulatory bodies details the study conduct. It is inevitable in a complex study with human participants that what occurs in practice will not be fully in accordance with the planned study in absolutely every aspect. Some instances of discrepancy are of no meaningful interest. Other such instances are substantial and undesirable and efforts should be made so that repetitions are avoided as a far as possible. Deviations from the protocol may pose a threat to the scientific credibility of the study and/or impact patient safety. A useful and common term to categorize such events is 'protocol deviations'. The term 'serious breach (of GCP or the protocol)' in the UK and EU is also used for more serious events which are considered to be 'likely to affect to a significant degree the safety or physical or mental integrity of the participants, or the scientific value of the trial' (6,7). It is important to consider what might occur during the study set up to be clear about what is a protocol deviation and what is not. It needs to be clarified what would not be ideal but not against the protocol, what would constitute a deviation but not one of concern, and what would constitute a deviation from the protocol of concern. The last group are sometimes referred to as 'important' or 'major' protocol deviations; they might also constitute a serious breach of the protocol in the UK and EU setting. The term 'protocol violations' is sometimes used to generally refer to more serious events where the protocol has not been followed up though with varying definitions. The source of such occurrences may be the action of a participant, study centre or trial office staff, investigators, and/or sponsor's actions. An example of a protocol deviation, which is also a serious breach, would be a clinical trial participant receiving the wrong dose of an IMP, or an IMP used after its expiry date. In contrast, the failure to complete part of the intended data collection at a study visit could be a protocol deviation which does not meet the criteria for a serious breach nor be considered 'important' as a one-off. For example, the staff member may in error have only gone through three of four forms to be completed.

Depending upon the event that has occurred and its nature, immediate action may be needed. This could be in order to protect the participants' safety, train staff to avoid future occurrences, and inform relevant bodies (e.g. sponsor, ethics committee, and regulatory bodies). Having an up-to-date list of protocol deviations is important so that recurring events can be detected early and further remedial action taken. A 'corrective and preventive action plan' may be needed to resolve a compliance issue, and help prevent future occurrences of the same kind. The first step is to investigate to fully understand what has occurred and the underlying causes. After this, the severity and impact need to be considered. This includes assessing if it is a one-off instance or one of a number of related occurrences. A key consideration is whether there are any broader implications across the clinical trial (e.g. other study centres). Potentially, other clinical trials being conducted by the same groups may similarly need some adjustment to a process (overall or at a specific site). How urgently any adjustment needs to be made also needs to be considered. Following this, corrective action (addressing the current instances, e.g. confirming what is permissible and how affect data should be used) can be developed. Furthermore, preventative action (consideration of changes in processes including additional checks, and any staff training needs) in order to mitigate and ideally preclude the possibility of a future occurrence can be identified. An example might be an additional check of a form at the time of data entry to confirm everything has been documented correctly and actions are appropriate.

Recruitment, recruitment, and recruitment

The challenges of recruiting well

Despite all the careful planning, and prior experience of running clinical trials that can help avoid many pitfalls, the initial part of the recruitment period of a clinical trial is often very challenging. Reviews of trials from leading UK publicly funded trial schemes found a third or more studies required extensions to the planned recruitment period and ultimately only around 40–50% recruited to the original recruitment target (8,9). Industry trials which tend to have more funding may suffer less in this regard yet they too are far from immune to recruitment problems (10). The problem has been nicely summed up in 'Lasanga's law' whereby 'the number of participants actually available for recruitment in a study usually turns out to be much lower than estimated in advance' (11). Muench made the point more starkly by suggesting 'in order to be realistic, the number of cases promised in any clinical study must be divided by a factor of at least ten' (12). Poor recruitment leads to longer study conduct, and greater overall cost. In the worst case it may led to the study being stopped prematurely as there is no realistic hope of the study completing to plan, or even having sufficient added value to warrant continuing. Given the challenges, a separate study called a feasibility study or pilot trial may be carried out prior to the full clinical trial. This could be in order to learn on a small scale whether the study is likely to be 'feasible'. Alternatively, the general process could be tested in a small number of centres to understand what might need to be changed, and possibly collect some relevant data on eligibility, recruitment, or retention of participants.

Recruitment model

A key distinction can be made between two recruitment models and how recruitment will run. First, for some clinical trials, there is an existing pool of potential participants who meet at least some of the key inclusion criteria and may have indicated interest in being involved in a clinical trial. For example, a register of health volunteers interested in phase 1 trial participation, or patients with a long-term condition interested in research study participation. The second, and more common, model is where the clinical trial recruits opportunistically over time as individuals become and are identified as potentially eligible for the trial. For example, a disease is identified in the individual which requires treatment, such as a diagnosis of breast cancer. Alternatively, a previous treatment is deemed to have failed and further treatment is needed. First-line therapy for breast cancer has not been successful. Clinical trials recruiting under the first model are in principle much easier to recruit to as long as the pool from which individuals are approached is sufficiently large to recruit enough participants for the clinical trial. The second model can be challenging even when there will be more than sufficient potential patients. Such individuals still need to be identified at the right time for trial participation, and often the window for doing so is quite short. This is particularly true in emergency care, but is also the case for many other conditions where individuals need to be identified to allow them to be approached about the study. For example, suitable patients in a colorectal clinic may need to identified prior to the clinic in order to be ready (e.g. have the right member of staff present) to assess their suitability for a clinical trial of two surgical approaches, and approach them at the appropriate point in the care pathway.

The unpredictability of trial recruitment

A variety of factors are known to have a bearing upon the ease of recruitment (8,13). These include whether the treatments are available outside of the clinical trial, the nature of the intervention and control treatments and associated risks, whether the condition of interest is common or rare, and if it is a transitory or chronic condition, and the setting of recruitment. Nevertheless, actual recruitment is remarkably hard to predict even at the best of times. Unforeseen events, due to factors outside of the clinical trial, can play a large part, the most extreme in recent times being the impact of the COVID-19 pandemic which has had a chilling effect on trial recruitment across a vast array of clinical trials. Figure 8.1 shows the actual recruitment versus predicted for two phase 3 clinical trials. The hope is for actual recruitment as shown in Figure 8.1a where the target recruitment rate was not only met but exceeded. In this case, the target sample size was met 7 months ahead of schedule. However, much more typical of recruitment to phase 3 clinical trials is the delayed start shown in Figure 8.1b where set-up and receipt of all necessary approvals and supplies resulted in a substantial delay in the start of recruitment. Even after adjusting the original recruitment schedule for this delay, recruitment failed to meet expectations. In this trial, there was also a period with no recruitment due to

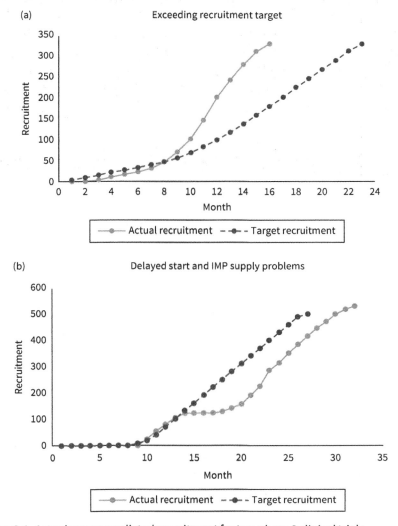

Figure 8.1 Actual versus predicted recruitment for two phase 3 clinical trials.

problems with the drug (IMP) supply. The target sample size was eventually reached though several months later than originally hoped.

Recruitment of participants is often where the impact of multiple problems within a clinical trial become most apparent. However, low recruitment (compared to what was expected) is often a symptom of issues in the study design or set-up with the main underlying problem being elsewhere (e.g. misspecification of the appropriate population for a phase 3 clinical trial which becomes apparent when the process is implemented in clinical practice). In the protocol, the number of study centres and anticipated recruitment period will have been specified along with the anticipated timelines. Contrasting this with the actual recruitment, both overall and by centre, can be a sobering experience for the trial team and investigators. Predicted recruitment levels tend to be overly optimistic, sometimes chronically so. While statistical models to predict recruitment based upon the current recruitment levels have been proposed, most clinical trial teams tend to use relatively simple methods to predict future prediction (14,15). Some common influencing factors can be identified to explain variations within and between centres. These include the centre's catchment area for potential participants, the impact of holidays (on potential participant numbers and centres' capacity to recruit), local investigator engagement, and centre attributes (location and services provided), among others factors. Seasonality can also play a part over the course of a calendar year (e.g. a trial looking at treatment for influenza needs to reflect the influenza season which is generally in October to April in the UK though this varies year to year, and will be different for other countries). However, as the examples in Figure 8.1 show, all such approaches are at best a guide. Unforeseen circumstances can come into play with the COVID-19 pandemic having brought many trials' recruitment to a standstill (indeed recruitment to some trials never recovered). Thankfully, unanticipated events that impact recruitment are usually more area specific, and short-term in nature, than the COVID-19 pandemic. Examples include the initiation of a new clinical trial in the same population competing for the participants, or the illness of the PI at a well-recruiting study centre.

Centre recruitment

Along with the overall recruitment, the number of study centres open for recruitment is also a useful indicator of progress. While centres will contribute to varying degrees, to an extent recruitment is a simple numbers game where more centres lead to more potential recruits, which in turn should ultimately result in more trial participants. This should be true even where there are substantial impediments to recruitment. However, centre initiation is a time-consuming task. Clinical trials will typically initially open with a subset of centres in the very early phase (often the one associated with the chief investigator) before bringing in other centres over time, often in waves. Data on past performance of recruiting centres in previous clinical trials can be used to aid selection of centres to approach about participating in a new clinical trial (16). Typically, a small number of centres contribute disproportionally, and a substantial number of centres will often recruit few or even no participants (this is usually true for both industry- and investigator-led studies) (16,17). A rate of one participant recruited per month per centre is not uncommon (18). 'Site fatigue', where recruitment to a clinical trial tapers off over time when a centre has been recruiting to a clinical trial for a long time, is not uncommon. Depending upon the specifics of the eligibility criteria, depletion of the local pool of potential participants might also contribute to slower recruitment over time. Assessment of centres' feasibility prior to initiation can help identify some problems in advance, and it can also clarify which centres may be more likely to be a better fit for the clinical trial (16). Comparison of the recruitment log between centres can give insights into engagement with the trial, and where problems may be arising. Differences in the number of reported eligible participants and the number screened can identify potential areas to clarify. However, the overall proportion of eligible participants who consent can vary greatly depending upon the trial design, population of interest, recruitment and consent processes implemented, and centre processes (8). Inactive centres which are open but not recruiting are a burden upon the trial office and local staff. Therefore, in some cases, closing centres early may be the appropriate thing to do for the overall benefit of the clinical trial.

Strategies to address low trial recruitment

Common approaches

Two main changes to clinical trial protocols can be implemented to address slow recruitment and increase the likelihood of reaching the target recruitment figure. These are the initiation of additional study centres, and extending the recruitment period. Often both are adopted together. Sometimes, a legitimate reduction in the sample size may be made (e.g. as imprecision of the primary outcome is less than anticipated and accounted for in the sample size, see Chapter 5) to at least partially resolve the issue. However, beyond the two overarching approaches, a wide variety of strategies are implemented to boost

Table 8.2 Most commonly reported strategies to improve recruitment

Strategy
Newsletters/mail shots/flyers (to clinical staff and/or patients)
Regular visits/phone calls to wards/centres/practices
Posters/information leaflets in clinics/wards/notes
Inclusion criteria changed/protocol amended
Presentations to appropriate groups (e.g. at consultant meetings/community-based physiotherapists, etc.)
Resource manual for centre staff/trained staff in disease area/procedures being investigated/role play exercises/study day/workshops for recruiters
Advertisement/articles in newspapers/journals; radio interviews
Presentations at national/international meetings
Employ extra staff
Investigator/recruiting staff meetings
Training/information videos
Incentives for recruiters (e.g. prize draw, chocolates, etc.)
Trial material revised/simplified/customized for specific centres
Visits to centres by principal investigators/senior members of study group
Repeated contact by phone/letter to individuals/centres
Increased/changed time points when information provided to potential participants
Supportive statements from opinion leaders

recruitment to the study (Table 8.2) (9). What will work well for a particular clinical trial may not work so well for another. Simplifications, and tailoring to the specific centres, of trial materials and processes, and maintaining regular contact with centres tend to be productive strategies. The support of clinical bodies may help with awareness and perceptions of the trial among potential investigators, and increased financial support (if possible) may remove some local barriers. There is surprisingly little research evidence on the value of these strategies (19) and this partly reflects the willingness to try multiple strategies at once to address recruitment difficulties (20,21). Happily, this is an area of clinical trial research with burgeoning interest. This perhaps reflects the increased challenges faced in this regard in conducting clinical trials over the last 20–30 years and decreasing sample sizes (22).

Approaching participants

A well-considered, practical, and timely process of approaching prospective participants about participating in the study, and consenting (or equivalent) is vital to healthy recruitment to a clinical trial. Problems with recruitment often relate to the failure to identify potential participants in a timely manner. They need to be approached at the point when participation in the trial is most sensible and convenient to them to take part (or for someone else to decide about participation where appropriate). Changes to the timing of the approach, who approaches the potential participant, or the manner in which it is done can lead to increased participation and improved overall recruitment. A process of informed consent given by the trial participant is the normal requirement for clinical trial participation, though as noted in Chapter 6 there are some exceptions. In some situations, the participant may not be able to consent (i.e. they lack the capacity to do so), and another individual may make the decision regarding their participation (e.g. parent or medical doctor). The participant (or alternatively, where they do not have capacity, a designated individual) needs to be provided with sufficient information about the study in a way that they can understand. They need to know what participation entails; this includes any associated risks and obligations on them (e.g. medical tests and assessments, and collection of their data). The consent given by an individual must also be voluntary and ongoing with the possibility of changing (i.e. reducing or rescinding completely) this consent. How the clinical trial is verbally presented (i.e. lack of clarity and inaccuracy or omission in stating fully what is known) by the trial staff conducting the approach to a potential participant can be a contributing factor to low recruitment rates. For example, the lack of equipoise between intervention and control treatments can lead to a lower level of consent as the individual's decision can be influenced by the recruiter (21). Low recruitment per se does not indicate the consent process is inadequate, as even after optimizing, recruitment may stay persistently low. However, going through such a process of evaluation can reveal unintended and unnecessary barriers. It may also identify ways in which study processes and the design could be modified to make it more appealing to potential participants. Thus, this could lead to modification to study documentation and requiring approval for a protocol amendment and related changes. Alternatively, such an assessment of the recruitment and consent processes may confirm the need to cease the study due to its infeasibility as designed. It is worth noting that a later clinical trial might succeed even though one seeking to address a very similar research question has failed to successfully recruit. The circumstances and differences in trial design might make it possible at another time even if it was not previously (23,24). Therefore, each trial needs to be considered in its own right when it comes to recruitment.

Retaining trial participants

While recruitment of participants is the hardest task faced when conducting clinical trials, it is by no means the only critical one. Retaining participants in the study (to prevent the loss of key data) is also vital. The loss of a participant from the clinical trial does not just mean that the participant's data are not available (i.e. as if they were not involved in the study). It is somewhat worse in that it has a detrimental impact upon the study's (statistical and ultimately scientific) value. Therefore, achieving good retention of participants to completion of a trial's follow-up is a key aspect of a high-quality clinical trial. Reviews of UK studies funded by leading governmental sources suggest 10% of participants without primary outcome data in an RCT is the norm and a trial having a level of 20% and above is not uncommon (8). As noted in Chapter 7, changes to a participant's consent (e.g. they may wish to 'withdraw' from the study) need to be carefully understood. A release from the more onerous elements of study participation may be what a participant wants as opposed to complete cessation of any involvement. They may not wish to cease future data collection related to them which does not include their involvement, only that they will not have to attend further study visits, or complete more forms. Often though participants may drift away from active participation in longer running studies. Where the study involvement requires multiple visits and completion of forms and questionnaire over months and years, it can be very difficult to maintain engagement. To some extent this drift may also be reflected in higher levels of changes to participant consent (25). Robust evidence pointing to effective strategies to improve retention is also lacking (26). Anecdotally, good communication and easily completed CRFs or equivalents are widely thought to be key (20,27). Careful monitoring of trial data, including return of key forms, and of changes in consent, will often be the first signs of an issue with how the clinical trial is being run and the demands upon participants. Greater engagement with participants (e.g. trial updates via newsletters and emails), clearer and easier to complete documentation, and telephone follow-up are common strategies to address low retention levels. The more drastic step, but sometime necessary one, of shortening of data collection to focus upon the most important data has also been used. For example, by removing information of secondary value, or collecting only a limited amount if the initial approach is not successful, a participant may be happy to provide this more limited set of information. Other strategies that have been used include monetary incentives, along with personalizing the approach and allowing more flexibility in how the form is return (e.g. postal or electronic, or via phone).

Data collection strategies

The clinical trial's data collection strategy which was considered in Chapter 7 needs to take into account not only providing a way in which in which the data can be returned but one by which the return of data is made straightforward. Participants and study centre staff often have many competing demands for their attention and time. Mechanisms of reminding them, politely, often pay dividends—as does anything that makes return of data easier (e.g. prepaid and addressed envelopes or automatic links to data entry). Example approaches that might be used in a clinical trial are given in Table 8.3. Two of the more common ways in which data are collected in most clinical trials, attendance at clinic and via form sent to participants by post, are covered. A

Table 8.3 Example retention strategies for common data collection methods

Data collection mode	Time points	Completed by	Approach to maximize return
Clinic visit where CRF is completed	3 and 6 months	Site staff	• Automated email to centres reminding them of visit and the need to schedule with participant • Request notification from centres of planned visit dates • Allow 1 month for return of form after time point • Email a report to centres every 6 weeks that lists missing CRFs • Ad hoc contact from trial office to centres regarding CRF return
Postal questionnaire	3, 6, and 12 months	Participant	• Questionnaires will be posted 3 days before follow-up is due • Participants will have 10 days to complete the questionnaire (to account for postage for those completing on paper) • First reminder will be sent 11 days after questionnaire is due • If still no response, phone calls will be used to obtain primary outcome • Review of return rates monthly by Trial Management Group in the first instance

common feature is not to rely on a single instance for completion as further approaches can lead to a substantially higher return level.

Close out and the 'end' of the trial

The last act of the clinical trial from a regulatory perspective is the close out (or completion) of the study. This is by no means the end of the clinical trial in a scientific sense (indeed data from the study may be used many years later) but it does mark completion of principle regulatory duties of the sponsor and the investigators, and the end of active regulatory oversight (e.g. cessation of annual safety reporting). A formal notice of the end of the study (from the regulatory perspective) will be required by the relevant regulatory bodies (e.g. ethics committee, and MHRA for a CTIMP in the UK). Final reports may also need to be submitted to regulatory bodies within a specified timeframe of the stated end of the trial. Prior to this, all study centres and potentially other bodies will need to have been notified when recruitment to the study formally ceased. The exact definition of the formal regulatory 'end of the trial' should be stated in the trial protocol but needs to encompass recruitment, data collection, processing and cleaning to the point of database closure as it pertains to the main objectives of the clinical trials. Trial close out is the process of preparing for and implementing the completion of the study. Closing-out a clinical trial operates at two levels. First, each study centre needs to be closed once relevant data collection and cleaning is complete. Study IMP, materials, and equipment will need to be dealt with appropriately. Second, as a whole study the study can be closed but only once the process has been completed for all study centres. All safety events will need to have been reviewed, clarified and classified appropriately prior to study closure. The finalised TMF will need to contain all the relevant documentation (electronic and paper), and this will need to be archived according to institutional, funder and regulatory authority bodies requirements. The trial registry entry (see Chapter 10) should be updated accordingly to report the results once available, indeed this may be a legal requirement (e.g. in the US and the EU). Other forms of dissemination (Chapter 10) may be ongoing for some time after the regulatory end and closer out of the study.

Summary

Running a clinical trial is where the aspirations of the scientific design meet the constraints of regulation, staffing resources, patient population, and other practical realities. Careful study set-up can prevent many problems though it should be anticipated that issues will arise when running the clinical trial which will need to be addressed. Recruitment and retention levels are the hard indicators of the progress of the clinical trial but hidden beneath them are many contributing factors. Some modification to the protocol should be expected and implemented carefully and rapidly. Without due monitoring, quick action is difficult, and a slowly progressing but completable clinical trial can become another prematurely stopped trial. Investigator and trial team persistence and resilience are key to a successful trial, along with making use of available support, and harnessing the know-how of those who have been through it before.

References

1. Finney DJ. An international drug safeguard plan. Journal of Chronic Diseases. 1964;17:565–81.
2. Lane JA, Gamble C, Cragg WJ, Tembo D, Sydes MR. A third trial oversight committee: functions, benefits and issues. Clinical Trials. 2020;17(1):106–12.
3. Norman JE, Norrie J, Maclennan G, Cooper D, Whyte S, Cunningham Burley S, et al. Open randomised trial of the (Arabin) pessary to prevent preterm birth in twin pregnancy with health economics and acceptability: STOPPIT-2—a study protocol. BMJ Open. 2018;8(12):e026430.
4. International Council for Harmonisation of Technical Requirements for Pharmaceuticals for Human Use (ICH). Integrated addendum to ICH E6(R1): guideline for good clinical practice E6(R2). 2006. Available from: https://database.ich.org/sites/default/files/E6_R2_Addendum.pdf
5. Legislation.gov.uk. The Medicines for Human Use (Clinical Trials) Regulations 2004. 2004. Available from: https://www.legislation.gov.uk/uksi/2004/1031/contents/made
6. Medicines and Healthcare products Regulatory Agency. Guidance for the notification of serious breaches of GCP or the trial protocol. Version 6. 2020. Available from: https://assets.publishing.service.gov.uk/government/uploads/system/uploads/attachment_data/file/905577/Guidance_for_the_Notification_of_Serious_Breaches_of_GCP_or_the_Trial_Protocol_Version_6__08_Jul_2020.pdf
7. European Medicines Agency. Guideline for the notification of serious breaches of Regulation (EU) No 536/2014 or the clinical trial protocol. 2017. Available from: https://www.ema.europa.eu/en/documents/scientific-guideline/guideline-notification-serious-breaches-regulation-eu-no-536/2014-clinical-trial-protocol_en.pdf
8. Walters SJ, Bonacho Dos Anjos Henriques-Cadby I, Bortolami O, Flight L, Hind D, Jacques RM, et al. Recruitment and retention of participants in randomised controlled trials: a review of trials funded and published by the United Kingdom Health Technology Assessment Programme. BMJ Open. 2017;7(3):e015276.
9. McDonald AM, Knight RC, Campbell MK, Entwistle VA, Grant AM, Cook JA, et al. What influences recruitment to randomised controlled trials? A review of trials funded by two UK funding agencies. Trials. 2006;7:9.
10. Kasenda B, von Elm E, You J, Blümle A, Tomonaga Y, Saccilotto R, et al. Prevalence, characteristics, and publication of discontinued randomized trials. JAMA. 2014;311(10):1045–51.

11. Knottnerus JA, Tugwell P. Prevention of premature trial discontinuation: how to counter Lasagna's law. Journal of Clinical Epidemiology. 2016;80:1–2.
12. Cooper CL, Hind D, Duncan R, Walters S, Lartey A, Lee E, et al. A rapid review indicated higher recruitment rates in treatment trials than in prevention trials. Journal of Clinical Epidemiology. 2015;68(3):347–54.
13. Cook JA, Ramsay CR, Norrie J. Recruitment to publicly funded trials—are surgical trials really different? Contemporary Clinical Trials. 2008;29(5):631–4.
14. Urbas S, Sherlock C, Metcalfe P. Interim recruitment prediction for multi-center clinical trials. Biostatistics. 2022;23(2):485–506.
15. Carter RE, Sonne SC, Brady KT. Practical considerations for estimating clinical trial accrual periods: application to a multi-center effectiveness study. BMC Medical Research Methodology. 2005;5(1):11.
16. Laaksonen N, Bengtström M, Axelin A, Blomster J, Scheinin M, Huupponen R. Clinical trial site identification practices and the use of electronic health records in feasibility evaluations: an interview study in the Nordic countries. Clinical Trials. 2021;18(6):724–31.
17. Anisimov VV, Fedorov VV. Modelling, prediction and adaptive adjustment of recruitment in multicentre trials. Statistics in Medicine. 2007;26(27):4958–75.
18. Jacques RM, Ahmed R, Harper J, Ranjan A, Saeed I, Simpson RM, Walters SJ. Recruitment, consent and retention of participants in randomised controlled trials: a review of trials published in the National Institute for Health Research (NIHR) Journals Library (1997–2020). BMJ Open. 2022 Feb 14;12(2):e059230. doi: 10.1136/bmjopen-2021-059230. PMID: 35165116; PMCID: PMC8845327.
19. Treweek S, Pitkethly M, Cook J, Fraser C, Mitchell E, Sullivan F, et al. Strategies to improve recruitment to randomised trials. Cochrane Database of Systematic Reviews. 2018;2(2):MR000013.
20. Prescott RJ, Counsell CE, Gillespie WJ, Grant AM, Russell IT, Kiauka S, et al. Factors that limit the quality, number and progress of randomised controlled trials. Health Technology Assessment. 1999;3(20):1–143.
21. Donovan JL, Rooshenas L, Jepson M, Elliott D, Wade J, Avery K, et al. Optimising recruitment and informed consent in randomised controlled trials: the development and implementation of the Quintet Recruitment Intervention (QRI). Trials. 2016;17(1):283.
22. Gresham G, Meinert JL, Gresham AG, Meinert CL. Assessment of trends in the design, accrual, and completion of trials registered in ClinicalTrials.gov by sponsor type, 2000–2019. JAMA Network Open. 2020;3(8):e2014682.
23. Beard DJ, Davies LJ, Cook JA, MacLennan G, Price A, Kent S, et al. Total versus partial knee replacement in patients with medial compartment knee osteoarthritis: the TOPKAT RCT. Health Technology Assessment. 2020;24(20):1–98.
24. Beard DJ, Campbell MK, Blazeby JM, Carr AJ, Weijer C, Cuthbertson BH, et al. Considerations and methods for placebo controls in surgical trials (ASPIRE guidelines). Lancet. 2020;395(10226):828–38.
25. Whitham D, Turzanski J, Bradshaw L, Clarke M, Culliford L, Duley L, et al. Development of a standardised set of metrics for monitoring site performance in multicentre randomised trials: a Delphi study. Trials. 2018;19(1):557.
26. Gillies K, Kearney A, Keenan C, Treweek S, Hudson J, Brueton VC, et al. Strategies to improve retention in randomised trials. Cochrane Database of Systematic Reviews. 2021;3(3):MR000032.
27. Bertram S, Graham D, Kurland M, Pace W, Madison S, Yawn BP. Communication is the key to success in pragmatic clinical trials in Practice-based Research Networks (PBRNs). Journal of the American Board of Family Medicine: JABFM. 2013;26(5):571–8.

9
Analysing a clinical trial

A p-value is no substitute for a brain.

Gregg Stone and Stuart Pocock, 2010 (1)

Basic principles of statistical analyses of randomized trials

With the notable exception of some phase 1 clinical trials, the key strength of the statistical analysis of a clinical trial lies in its controlled nature; that is, there is a natural, concurrent, and comparable reference group to compare the treatment group's data to. In this chapter we will focus on the basic principles for conducting the analysis of an RCT. Here there is, by definition, always a control group. We will also mainly focus on the standard trial design when applying methods of statistical analysis given it is by far the most common design used and also to avoid further complexity. This chapter will not be able to cover the basics of medical statistics. Any reader wishing to do so is encouraged to read one of many excellent introductions to medical statistics to understand the basics of statistical analysis (2,3). Here we will follow a frequentist (i.e. conventional) approach to statistical analysis (see below for further discussion of this). The statistical analysis should have already been considered to some degree when designing the study (particularly how the primary outcome and key secondary outcomes are going to be analysed). A trial protocol will have a summary of the intended statistical analysis and the corresponding strategy and main methods planned to be used. The full statistical analysis strategy should be fleshed out prior to the point where the analysis needs to be conducted. When we first think of how to statistically analyse data, it is natural to want to jump to the choice of statistical analysis methods. However, before we consider this and related issues, we begin with seven key principles of the statistical analyses of randomized trials.

Principle one—the statistical analysis should reflect the design

The first and most basic principle to begin with is that the main statistical analysis should reflect the clinical trial design. For an RCT, it should therefore be a comparison *between* the randomized groups. This is the case even if no formal statistical test is made, and only an informal or descriptive analysis is done. It should be made with reference to the randomized groups. It is the randomized groups which we expect to be the same except for the treatment received (if the trial is well conducted, and all things being equal). We therefore want the main analysis to compare the randomized groups. It may surprise some readers that RCTs are sometimes analysed as if they were not comparative studies yet this has been done (4). For a standard trial design with simple (1:1) randomization, if we use an analysis that compares the two randomized groups we are on safe ground. If another clinical trial design has been used, the preferable analysis is one that correspondingly reflects the specifics of the trial design we have adopted.

There are three further aspects of trial design which we would to take in account in developing our analysis strategy:

1. First, if we use an alternative trial design we will need to address this in our analysis strategy. For example, if we have a three-arm RCT we need to think about how our analysis will reflect this and the potential for differences in any of the three treatment groups. Typically, this will mean analyses which compare pairs of treatment as this will likely be needed to address the study objectives. An overall comparison, or some comparison of subsets of combinations of groups, may also be appropriate. The approach needs to be thought through and mapped to the main research question and study objectives.

2. Second, if we have incorporated any variables in our randomization algorithm we will want to use a statistical analysis method which adjusts for them. We need to do this otherwise the analysis result will be too imprecise (reflected in the width of the confidence interval and the corresponding p-value for the comparison) (5).

3. Third, if we are proposing to collect data more than once for our outcome, or over a period of time (e.g. morality over 2 years), we need to address this in our analysis strategy. There are various ways we can do so. We could pick a single time point up to which we think it is most

important to compare the outcome at. Alternatively, we could use an analysis method that utilizes all the available data such as multiple outcome time points or when the events of interest occurred.

As for most 'rules' there are exceptions or scenarios where fully reflecting the design in the analysis is difficult or even suboptimal. However, as a general rule, as the trial is designed, so it should be analysed. It is worth noting that statistical analyses are shaped (and constrained) by the study design. Crudely put, we can only analyse data that have been collected. As such, we cannot rectify critical design errors with more sophisticated statistical analyses. We can only try to attenuate the impact of them.

Principle two—include all individuals randomized in the analysis

The second key principle is that we want to include all of the individuals who were randomized in the corresponding analysis treatment groups. Failing to do so will, to some degree, dilute the statistical benefits of randomization. Data from clinical trials can later be used for a variety of other useful analyses. Those which are faithful to the design will recognize the comparative nature of the study design as we have considered above. For example, a systematic review of RCTs should be meta-analysed in a way that recognizes the design of the study from which the data came from. Furthermore, the analysis should typically acknowledge the allocated group irrespective of what occurs in terms of receipt of treatment. Hopefully there will be no 'non-compliance' or failure to receive the allocated treatment as intended (e.g. a participant does not take the allocated drug tablets). Nevertheless, even if/when it does occur, the default main analysis, except in the most exceptional circumstances, should group the data 'as randomized'. Commonly, the phase 'intention to treat' is used to clarify the data has been grouped in the analysis in this way, and also whose data is included in each analysis group. Grouping data as randomised corresponds to the conventional analytic target (implicit in the use of standard analyses) of testing for a difference between the randomised groups. As per principle one the corresponding analysis will then reflect the trial design. This is sometimes referred to as an intention to treat analysis. Due to withdrawals, and missing data it may not be feasible to include data for all randomised participants in the analysis. However, we should seek to include as far as possible data from all individuals (or whatever unit was allocated) randomised in the analysis, minimise exclusions, and recognise that our analysis strategy needs to respect the random allocation.

Principle three—be clear about the analytic aim of the analysis

The third principle is to be clear about the analytic aim of the analysis of each outcome. Beyond the mere grouping of the data, we need to decide how exactly we will numerically compare the randomised groups for each outcome. This decision has at times wrongly only been made implicitly by choosing the analysis method according to the data available and reporting what the method provides by default. We should instead think about this upfront and be clear about what we are seeking to do. Accordingly, we might state for a continuous outcome we are interested the average treatment effect (the ATE as is it is often abbreviated to) on those randomised. The ATE is defined as the difference between the mean outcome values in the respective randomised groups (i.e. mean of the intervention group outcome values minus the mean of the control group outcome values). We conveniently can view the ATE as the causal effect of the treatment choice (as delivered in the randomised trial). For a standard RCT, the ATE can be calculated, simply as the mean difference between the outcome in the randomised groups: a difference in the means of intervention group ($\bar{y}_I$) and the control group ($\bar{y}_C$) observations, that is, $\bar{y}_I - \bar{y}_C$.

Given a standard trial design with 1:1 allocation and a reasonable sample size, the mean difference can be then be estimated unbiasedly and robustly, with associated uncertainty using standard methods (such as linear regression) (6). Note we are estimating the same quantity we made an assumption about in the sample size for a continuous outcome in Chapter 5 (δ as it appears in formula 5.1). For other outcome types (e.g. binary or time to event), the choice of analysis method and the specifics of its application (especially regarding model adjustment for prognostic factors) requires more care, and typically imply further assumptions particularly using regression models (5). Nevertheless, whatever outcome we have and whatever method we choose to analyse it, we should be clear about what we are seeking to estimate. The corresponding analytic application for other trial designs may require some modification of the approach. For a cluster trial where we allocate clusters and not individuals, we can compare the data from the clusters that were randomized to each treatment. Furthermore, we will want to include in the analysis data for all relevant individuals within these clusters (for a cluster trial who they are may not be obvious like in a standard RCT). We can use a model which allows for the clustering of data (due to the cluster random- isation) to be accounted for (e.g. a multilevel model) (2). It is worth noting in passing that where a non-inferiority or equivalence trial is being analysed, the pre-eminence of an intention-to-treat analysis is less clear (see Chapter 2 for discussion of superiority, non-inferiority, and equivalence). The most appropriate way to handle non-compliance is less clear in this setting (as non- compliance to random allocation tends to lead to diluting any difference between the groups i.e. making the groups appear more similar). For non- inferiority or equivalence trials, a per-protocol analysis which focuses on the data from participants who complied with the treatment protocol as allocated is very commonly conducted as well as an 'as randomized'-based analysis. We will consider other, potentially superior analyses that address non-compliance later in the chapter.

Principle four—use outcome data in a consistent and fair manner

A fouth key principle is that the outcomes we wish to compare between the groups need to have been collected in a consistent and fair manner across the groups. This might at first seem more an issue for data collection and not the statistical analysis. Indeed, data collection processes can and should be designed and implemented in order to collect such data fairly. However, by analysing the data we are acting as if it is reasonable to compare it. Therefore, it is important to pause before analysing it to consider whether this is indeed the case. For example, we could have an outcome that can only occur in one of the randomized groups (e.g. we could collect data on surgical complica- tions in an RCT comparing surgery and a medical treatment). Here we do not have a coherent analysis to compare the outcome between the groups even though we can carry out a statistical test and get a result. This is not to say that collection of data on surgical complications and related treatments is irrelevant in our example. Only that it cannot be an outcome for which we compare between these randomized groups in any statistically meaningful way. Instead, we could usefully quantify it for the relevant treatment group (e.g. the surgery group in our example). Or we could define an outcome that allows for similar events in both groups (e.g. the need for further treatment). Either way, care in interpretation is needed due to the difference in the nature of the treatments.

Principle five—recognize that the observed outcome data has multiple causes

A fifth principle is that we need to analyse the data and interpret them recognizing that outcomes vary between individuals for a variety for reasons. It is critical to understand that the results we observe *could* have occurred by chance no matter how apparently strong they are on initial viewing due to variation in outcome between patients. Such variation is inherent across patients and medical care. The observed result for each individual will have multiple factors that contribute to what we observe (e.g. genetics, general health, disease status, treatments received, and the study design). We need to anticipate this. Suppose we conducted an RCT to compare two treatments which work equally well. We will likely observe by chance that one of the treatments has numerically better outcome data than the other one when we compare the observed summary data for the two groups. Were we to be able to do the study again many times, we would get a variety of results (or better put, statistically, we call it a distribution). Typically, we are not in such a (statistically) luxurious situation of carrying out our studies multiple times. Indeed, we might find such an idea morally repugnant or at least a grossly inefficient use of resources. We therefore wish to conduct analyses of each clinical trial's data which account for this possibility of variation by chance. This will help us come to a view about how unusual or not our findings are. This is what a statistical analysis does by seeking to assess what is plausible given the observed data, and how unusual the observed values are. Commonly this is ultimately reflected in the analysis outputs such as a p-value or better still a confidence interval which provides a range of values which are consistent with the observed data given the analysis conducted.

Principle six—use analyses that quantify the magnitude of the effect and associated uncertainty

The sixth key principle is that analyses which quantify the magnitude of the effect and the corresponding uncertainty (e.g. expressed as a confidence interval) are to be preferred over statistical methods which only provide a formal statistical test (i.e. provide a p-value). Statistical methods are commonly used in medical research and also to analyse data from clinical trials that do not provide an estimate of the magnitude of effect (e.g. chi-squared tests). However, they are by themselves an unsatisfactory basis to summarize the results (7). The reason is irrespective as to whether the result is statistically significant or not; we are interested in the magnitude of effect that is plausible given the data and the chosen analysis. For example, if we found the risk of a side effect (e.g. headache) was lower in one group, we would naturally want to know by how much, particularly if this treatment is more unpleasant to receive (e.g. may cause nausea) than an alternative which has the higher risk of a headache. To be able to make a choice, we need to understand the magnitude of the observed difference (e.g. was it a 10% reduction in the risk or is it only 2%?). We also want to know how large or small a difference the data support (e.g. is as large as 20% and as small as 1% something that is plausible?). Recognition of this is one of the reasons for carrying out a sample size calculation. It should help ensure the study has a reasonable chance of being informative as we state what we are interested in finding. Correspondingly, we should follow through with this in the statistical analysis (not just whether there is evidence of a difference or not at the chosen significance level). We should use a statistical method that quantifies the magnitude of the effect, and the related uncertainty. Otherwise, we are leaving it up to the reader to calculate the magnitude of the treatment effect themselves and guess the level of imprecision.

Principle seven—statistical analyses should be planned

A seventh key principle of analysing RCTs is to recognize that the main analyses should be planned in advance. A key feature of clinical trials is they are planned experiments and this planning should extend to the statistical analysis. This does not mean no further analyses can be done which are not specified in advance, merely that the main ones should be specifiable, or where they are no longer appropriate, a justification should be provided. The sample size will typically have been calculated on a statistical basis implying a particular analysis method (or type of analysis) corresponding to the data expected to be available. The basic statistical analysis strategy should be summarized in the clinical trial's protocol and potentially any prior funding application. Increasingly a separate document called a statistical analysis plan (SAP for short) is used which is drafted and approved in advance of the key trial data analyses. Multiple analyses for the primary outcome and key secondary outcome may be planned. Additionally, how compliance and missing data are dealt with may lead to additional analyses. This should be covered as well as the basic statistical principles adopted such as the grouping of the data and the general statistical approach.

Different statistical analyses

Having considered the principles that should inform our analysis strategy, we now consider why different statistical analyses might be appropriate. Commonly there will be more than one statistical analysis of key outcomes, particularly the primary outcome of a randomized trial. Different analyses might lead to different results, both due to genuine differences between the analyses in what is being tested, and due to spurious 'signals' in the data. To address this, it is common to *pre-specify* (i.e. state before the analysis is conducted) what can be described as the main analysis of each outcome. Other analyses of interest known to be important before analysing the data can also be specified but viewed as being of a supporting nature to the interpretation of the primary outcome result. A common further analysis, which might be described as a 'sensitivity analysis', is where the same analysis is carried out but with additional adjustment for a key variable believed to be related to outcome. The International Stroke Trial (IST) RCT evaluated treatments for patients with acute ischaemic stroke. Age at baseline was thought likely to be related to chance of death, and therefore a further analysis adjusted for age given the main analysis did not (8). Alternatively, where there is reason to doubt one of the assumptions required by the method to be used for the main analysis (e.g. normality for linear regression), it would be natural to also conduct a further analysis which addressed this concern. This might require a different statistical analysis method which is not reliant on this assumption. We could plan for this in advance. Use of a different statistical analysis method can be described as a 'secondary analysis'. Particular care is needed when doing so and interpreting the results. Different statistical methods might imply a different, though superficially the same, comparison. For example, the 'non-parametric' Mann–Whitney U test is often used instead of an independent t-test due to concerns about the impact of non-normality. However, the t-test compares the mean between the treatment groups, whereas the Mann–Whitney U test compares the distributions (i.e. the shape as well as the location). If the result of a Mann–Whitney U test is significant this implies a difference in distributions, not just a difference in the location (e.g. median) between the groups. It is useful to note that each statistical method has different assumptions and properties. While statistical methods used appropriately will mostly agree, they will not always do so (9). It is therefore critical to pre-specify and report clearly which statistical analysis is the main one where more than one has been used.

Methods of analysis

Statistical framework

To statistically analyse outcome data from an RCT, we need to adopt a statistical approach. In this chapter we are following what might be described as a conventional (or frequentist) statistical approach to analysing clinical trials and RCTs (10). This is the approach to the analysing data which most readers will be familiar with if they have undergone ('suffered'/'enjoyed', delete as applicable) an introductory medical statistics course. The conventional approach is by far the most common statistical approach to analysing medical data and there are numerous excellent introductory texts for those looking to brush up on the basics (2). Like any approach it has its limitations, and indeed these stem from its strengths. This approach seeks to limit the number of assumptions made in order to analyse the data. It is also concerned primarily with the challenge posed by (sampling) variability. Other statistical approaches are possible, such as adopting a 'Bayesian' approach. In general, these are more flexible (in principle at least) but they are also more complex and time-consuming to use (2). While the application of such methods is becoming more common it is still used in only a small minority of clinical trials and RCTs. In general, the principles discussed here apply to the application of Bayesian methods. The focus here is not on the equations or the derivation of methods but the underlying statistical principles and the application of methods according to them. For example, credible intervals are the natural Bayesian equivalent of a confidence interval when seeking to quantify uncertainty about a parameter of interest (e.g. mean difference). If desired, a Bayesian 'p-value' (i.e. the probability under the posterior distribution) can be produced as an alternative to a p-value. Arguably this is a more useful direct value of interest related to our point of inference (e.g. is treatment A different from B?). The use of Bayesian methods is covered in depth elsewhere (2,11,12).

Choosing the statistical method

Beyond the general statistical framework, we are faced with an exceptionally large number of potential statistical analysis methods which could be used. Indeed, many have been used to analyse data from a clinical trial. Fortunately, in practice, there are a much smaller number of analysis methods that are commonly used. A handful of general rules can be applied to help us choose an appropriate method. First, the method should provide a result which addresses the relevant study objective. Second, an analysis method should be chosen in recognition of the data that is expected to be available. Note the intentional use of 'expected' versus 'to be collected' as not everything we may try to collect can realistically be expected for all participants. Third, statistical methods which require the least onerous assumptions to provide a valid analysis should be favoured unless there is a substantial benefit in terms of clarity from an alternative. In this chapter we are focusing on analysing data from RCTs. We will consider the analysis of a continuous outcome, a binary outcome, and also a time-to-event outcome. These are the same three outcome types we considered in Chapter 5 where we looked at how to carry out sample size calculations. Common statistical analysis methods for these outcome types will be used and applied to RCT data to illustrate their use.

Analysing a continuous outcome

We will consider data from a trial of two operations of knee surgery: total and partial knee replacement. Data from the TOPKAT trial are shown in Table 9.1 for the primary outcome, the OKS—a measure of knee function and pain. The OKS was measured at baseline and 5 years after randomization. Data were available for 233 and 231 participants in the partial knee replacement and total knee replacement randomized groups, respectively (13). The mean OKS in both groups were very similar at 5 years with group means of 38.0 and

Table 9.1 TOPKAT trial analyses of the Oxford Knee Score

Time point	OKS by randomized group						Statistical analysis		
	Partial knee replacement (N = 264)			Total knee replacement (N = 264)				Mean difference (95% CI)	P-value
	n	mean	SD	n	mean	SD			
Baseline	264	18.8	7.0	264	19.0	7.2		N/A	
5 years	233	38.0	10.1	231	37.0	10.6	Unadjusted[a]	1.0 (−0.9 to 2.9)	0.29
							Adjusted[b]	1.0 (−0.4 to 2.5)	0.16

CI, confidence interval; OKS, Oxford Knee Score; SD, standard deviation; N/A, not assessed.

[a] Unadjusted analysis using independent t-test. [b] Adjusted for age, sex, baseline OKS score, and surgeon delivering operation using linear regression. Surgeon was accounted for using cluster-robust variance estimation.

37.0. This reflects a substantial numerical increase from baseline (both groups had means of approximately 19.0 at baseline). The OKS ranges from 0 to 48 and can for convenience be analysed as if it were a continuous outcome. We can readily apply a linear regression model to estimate the mean difference between the two randomized groups given the standard RCT design. This respects principles one to five outlined above. We can do this without any adjustment for other factors (an 'unadjusted analysis'). This is equivalent to carrying out an independent t-test to compare the mean OKS between the two randomized groups (assuming common variance). We can calculate the mean difference by a simple subtraction with 38.0 minus 37.0, that is, the OKS was 1.0 point higher on average in the partial knee replacement group. However, to calculate the corresponding confidence interval and to calculate a p-value we need to do more work. Typically when analysing clinical trial data we use a statistical program to carry out the calculations automatically for us to avoid simple errors and for ease and speed. Doing so we find the 95% confidence interval for the mean difference is from −0.9 to 2.9 with a corresponding p-value of 0.29. Therefore, we do not have statistical evidence of a difference at the two-sided 5% significance level. This can also be seen in that the 95% confidence interval for the difference in means contain zero, that is, the interval contains the point where both groups have the same mean OKS value (i.e. no difference). The range of values in the interval are not that large roughly from an average difference of almost one in favour of total knee replacement to a difference of just under 3 points in favour of partial knee replacement.

However, this is not the full story as the trial used minimization to randomize participants to the intervention. The randomization controlled for the participant's sex, age, OKS at study entry, and also the surgical group involved in delivering the operation (13). As per key principle one above, we therefore would like an analysis that reflects these variables. Furthermore, adjusting for these variables may additionally provide a more precise result. The corresponding result was 1.0, 95% confidence interval (−0.4 to 2.5) providing a slightly narrower confidence interval. However, there was as before, no statistical evidence of a difference at the (two-sided) 5% level. Again, the confidence interval for the difference in means contains zero. The range of values consistent with the data suggesting at most a modest difference in favour of partial knee replacement (2.5 points) cannot be ruled out at this significance level. In others words, the analysis found no clear evidence of a difference in OKS between the groups. However, it did not rule out a small difference in favour of partial knee replacement. The possible difference in favour of total knee replacement within the interval though was only 0.4 which was considered likely to be of little clinical value.

Analysing a binary outcome

For our analysis of a binary outcome, we use data from the Learning Early about Peanut Allergy (LEAP) trial (14). It recruited 640 infants with severe eczema, egg allergy, or both, to receive either consumption or avoidance of peanuts until 60 months of age. Parents of the participants in the consumption group were supplied with peanut products for the infants to consume with three or four meals a week. For infants in the avoidance group, parents were requested to avoid giving them peanuts until they were 60 months old. The primary outcome was the proportion of participants with a peanut allergy at 60 months. Infants received a skin prick test (SPT) for peanut allergy at study entry (baseline). Two groups of infants were recruited to the study: those who had a negative SPT at study entry, and those who had a positive (but not too severe) SPT result at study entry. For simplicity, we focus on the result of the combined groups (both SPT-positive and -negative groups). The results for the 628 participants grouped according to the random allocation are given in Table 9.2. We can see there were 10 (3.2%) and 54 (17.2%) infants who were allergic in the consumption and avoidance groups, respectively. Obviously these appear to be quite different levels of peanut allergy.

When analysing a binary outcome, we have three common alternative measures that can be readily used to quantify the magnitude of the observed difference between the groups as we considered in Chapter 5. These are an OR, a RR, and/or a risk difference in the proportions (if we multiply the latter

Table 9.2 LEAP trial comparison of consumption versus no consumption analysis of allergic reaction

Time point	Allergy by randomized group						Statistical analysis		
	Consumption (randomized = 319)			Avoidance (randomized = 321)					
	n	N	%	n	N	%	Effect measure (95% CI)		P-value
60 months	10	314	3.2	54	314	17.2	Risk difference in percentages[a]	−14% (−19% to −9%)	N/A
							Odds ratio[b]	0.16 (0.08 to 0.32)	<0.001
							Risk ratio[c]	0.19 (0.10 to 0.36)	<0.001

CI, confidence interval; N/A, not assessed.

[a] Newcombe's method no. 10 (16). [b] Logistic regression. [c] Confidence interval method implemented in the cs command in Stata (17).

by 100 it can be presented as a percentage difference). Briefly, the OR is the odds (probability of an event divided by the probability of not having the event) in one of the groups divided by the odds in the other group. The RR is the risk (number of events divided by number of individuals in the group) in one group divided by the risk in the other group. The risk difference is the risk in one group minus the risk in the other group. Due to limited space, we do not consider in detail the definitions and merits of each in length and refer the reader to useful texts elsewhere (2,15,16). We will illustrate the three different results using a statistical analysis method which compares the respective effect size measure using the same data. We note in passing we would typically only use one of these effect size measures, and base our analysis strategy around methods which calculate it. Furthermore, to respect principle seven, we should plan this in advance and pre-specify what the main analysis is.

We now use a method to calculate an estimate of the OR, RR, and risk difference in turn using the data in Table 9.2. The risk difference in percentages is 14% lower in the consumption group. Using Newcombe's method no. 10 (17) to calculate the 95% confidence interval, we see that it is from −9% to −19%, that is, the percentage of allergy at 60 months could be between 9 and 19% lower in the consumption group. This method does not by default produce a corresponding p-value though one could be produced if desired. As before the inclusion or not of the null value (here 0%) indicates significance at the specified level (i.e. 2-sided 5% for a 95% confidence interval). If instead we wanted to calculate an OR, we could use logistic regression (with the randomized treatment group as the only independent variable) (2). We use a model with the randomized treatment group as the only explanatory variable in the model (i.e. an unadjusted analysis of the 'as randomized' groups). Doing so we get an OR of 0.16 with 95% confidence interval (0.08 to 0.32), that is, the point estimate is a 84% reduction in the odds in the consumption group. The corresponding confidence interval ranges from a 68% to a 92% reduction in the odds of a peanut allergy in the consumption group compared to the avoidance group. The corresponding p-value is less than 0.001 reflecting a very small chance of the data occurring by change if there was no difference between the groups (given the data observed and the method used). Similarly, if we wanted to calculate the RR we could do so using a suitable confidence interval method such as the one implemented in the cs command in Stata (18). Doing so we get a RR of 0.19 with 95% confidence interval (0.10 to 0.36). The corresponding p-value is again very small, less than 0.001. The result is an observed reduction of 81% in the risk of a peanut allergy in the consumption group. The confidence interval ranged from a 64% to a 90% reduction in the consumption group. Note the OR and RR here are quite similar though that does not need to be the case. If there had been a higher rate of allergy then the OR and the RR estimates would diverge.

Two points are particularly worth emphasizing. First, none of the three treatment effect measure (or any alternative) can be claimed to be clearly better than the other options. Of the three shown here, each has its own strengths. A risk difference in percentages is perhaps the easiest to understand but it is more difficult to adjust for than other variables in the statistical analysis (e.g. if we wanted to account for age at baseline or sex, etc.), and tends to require slightly more data to detect a difference. ORs are mathematically convenient to work with for statistical reasons beyond the scope of the book (19). Using logistic regression makes modelling easy to apply, but the least readily interpretable result of the three effect measures presented here. The RR arguably fall between the aforementioned two measures in terms of interpretability and convenience of analysis. Irrespective of which is used for a binary outcome, it is important to consider the findings in terms of what both the absolute (e.g. difference in percentages) and the relative effect is (e.g. change in risk). Second, all the analyses in Table 9.2 have in essence the same result, that the consumption group had a markedly lower level of peanut allergy at 60 months. However, there are minor differences between the results of the methods (aside from the obvious distinct way the treatment difference is expressed). Had the trial result been a borderline difference (in favour or either group), the three different analyses could have led to (nominally) different conclusions when judged on statistical significance alone.

Analysing a time-to-event outcome

We now consider the analysis of a time-to-event outcome. Here we use data from the IST trial (8). The trial adopted a 2 × 2 factorial trial design to allow it to look at two treatments in conjunction. For simplicity we focus only on the aspirin comparison and also on only one of the two primary outcomes: death within 14 days. We begin with analysing the data as a binary outcome in the same manner as above. The results are given in Table 9.3 according to the randomized groups. We can see there were 872 (9.0%) and 909 (9.4%) deaths in the aspirin and no aspirin groups, respectively, at 14 days. Obviously these are very similar values on the face of it, and any statistical test is unlikely to detect a difference. However, we do have a large study here and it is useful to clarify how close or not it is to meeting criteria for statistical significance (typically two-sided 5% level). We would like to know how certain (or not) we are about the possibility of a difference between the groups. We now use the same three statistical methods as in the LEAP trial example to calculate each in turn using the

Table 9.3 IST trial comparison of aspirin versus no aspirin analysis of death

Time point	Death by randomized group						Statistical analysis		
	Aspirin (randomized= 9720)			No aspirin (randomized = 9715)					
	n	N	%	n	N	%	Effect measure	(95% CI)	P-value
Day 14	872	9719	9.0	909	9714	9.4	Risk difference in percentages	0.4% (−1.2% to 0.4%)	N/A
Day 100	1854	9719	19.1	1795	9714	18.5	Odds ratio	0.95 (0.87 to 1.05)	0.35
							Risk ratio	0.96 (0.88 to 1.05)	0.35
							Hazard ratio	0.97 (0.91 to 1.03)	

Note: N/A, not assessed

data in Table 9.3. The risk difference at day 14 is 0.4% higher in the no aspirin group and using Newcombe's method (no. 10.) to calculate the 95% confidence interval we see that it is calculated to go from −1.2% to 0.4% (i.e. the percentage of death could be 1.2% lower in the aspirin group to 0.4% higher in the aspirin group). We get an OR for an event up to day 14 of 0.95 with 95% confidence interval (0.87 to 1.05), that is, a point estimate of 5% reduction in the odds of death in the aspirin group with a confidence interval ranging from 13% reduction to a 5% increase. The corresponding p-value is 0.35 reflecting the similarity in the estimated value. The calculated RR using the same method as for the LEAP example above is 0.96 with 95% confidence interval (0.88 to 1.05) with a p-value of 0.35; in other words, there is an observed reduction of 4% in the risk of death in the aspirin group with the confidence interval ranging from a 12% reduction in the aspirin group to a 5% increase in the aspirin group.

So far we have considered mortality as a binary outcome and analysed it accordingly. However, as we have the information relating to when death occurred, we have an alternative option which is to analyse the data as a time-to-event (or 'survival') outcome. The advantage is that if we know the outcome for participants over varying periods of time (i.e. not always exactly 14 days), we can include them for whatever period of time we do know their status. We will therefore use the data about deaths occurring within the first 100 days. We can graphically represent this as a Kaplan–Meier curve, one for each of the two randomized groups (Figure 9.1) (2). The curve shows how the probability

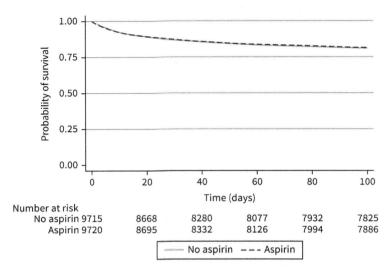

Figure 9.1 IST trial—Kaplan-Meier survival curve for death.

of survival changes over time as death occur. Time is subdivided into intervals (i.e. in this case as days) during which either an event occurs or does not occur for each individual. Data for each individual contribute for the period for which their status (death or not) is known. We plot one survival curve for each group so we can see if there are any obvious differences in the survival over time between the groups. Here we can see both groups have very similar survival curves and the relationship of one to the other appears to be consistent over time (i.e. there is no crossing of lines or change in the relative survival of one treatment to the other). The curves are also very smooth, reflecting the large number of participants with the full 100 days of follow-up. Implicitly it is assumed that all participants (whether 'censored' or not, i.e. whether they are known to have been alive for only part of the follow-up or the full 100 days) have the same risk of death. It is possible to compare the curve to test for a difference in the curves. A very commonly used test to do so is called the log-rank test which we came across in Chapter 5. Here we apply it and the resultant p-value is 0.29 which is not clearly significant at the two-sided 5% significance level. Therefore, there is no statistical evidence of a difference between the survival curves at this significance level. This is not surprising given the curves shown in Figure 9.1. However, it is desirable to be able to quantify the difference between the treatment groups and the uncertainty related to it. Furthermore, we may wish to use a method which will allow us to take into account other variables of interest.

A common statistical approach to analysing time-to-event data is to use a Cox proportional hazards model (2). We use a model with only the randomized treatment group as the only explanatory variable in the model (i.e. an unadjusted analysis of the 'as randomized' groups). Here the results are expressed as a ratio of the hazard (instant risk) of the event of interest (in our case death) at a specific point in time in the individuals for which the event has not occurred so far (i.e. are still alive at that point for our example). As discussed in Chapter 5, the term 'proportional hazards' in the name of the method refers to an assumption related to the pattern of survival which assumes the ratio of the 'hazards' (i.e. the risk of an event at a point in time given the participant has survived to that point) are consistent over time. If this is the case, then the hazards can be referred to as 'proportional' (20). The Cox proportional hazards model assumes this. However, if the hazards are not proportional, we either need to consider more complex analyses which deal with the changing of effect over time (e.g. time-varying effects which account for variables that may explain a change in the treatment's effect over time) (21) or we have to be more cautious in interpreting our results of our Cox proportional hazards model as it is an average of the actual ratio of the hazards over the follow-up period.

Given the shape of the survival curves we happily are not concerned about the assumption of proportional hazards being invalid. We can proceed with interpreting the findings. The results from this are again very similar to the previous analyses of death at day 14. The estimated HR is 0.97, 95% confidence interval (0.91 to 1.03), that is, hazards might range from 9% less to 3% more, so a very small hazard either way. As with the OR and RR, a value of 1.0 indicates the groups are estimated to have the same value (i.e. hazard). We can also quantify the survival at key points using the Kaplan–Meier curves. For example, survival at day 50 was estimated to be 85% and 84% in the aspirin and no aspirin groups. We could have picked any day of the curve and picked off the corresponding results. overall, there is no statistical evidence (at our chosen significance level) to conclude any difference in the risk of death between the randomized groups over time.

It is worth noting in passing that small differences are very difficult to detect but even harder to rule out. Despite including over 18,000 participants, our analysis cannot rule out the possibility of a 1% absolute decrease (or 12% relative reduction) in the risk of death at 14 days. The HR confidence interval included a 9% decrease to a 3% increase in the hazard. A frustrating and unintuitive aspect of statistics is that the more similar two groups are, the greater the amount of data that is required to demonstrate this. Finally, it is worth noting that such a small difference between treatments in most outcomes would often be considered clinically unimportant, or insufficient to justify using a more expensive or demanding to deliver treatment. Nevertheless, as we are taking about mortality here, a 1% absolute reduction in the risk (or 9% reduction in the hazard) cannot be readily discarded as of no interest. We now consider how we come to an overall conclusion for the study given we will likely have multiple outcomes with different results.

Coming to an overall conclusion

Having conducted our main analyses of the primary outcome we might consider the matter of the analysis closed. However, while we may have the main result of the clinical trial, we need to consider the results of the other (secondary) outcomes before we can have a final conclusion of the findings of the clinical trial, or RCT. We will typically have a number of further (secondary) outcomes in a clinical trial. We should plan how we will analyse these as well in our SAP. Each needs to be considered in turn regarding what an appropriate analysis approach would be in terms of the type of outcome and what is of key interest. Data on safety related to the treatments must also be considered. We now consider our three examples in turn again.

In the TOPKAT trial there were 14 secondary outcomes looking at other knee-specific outcomes, health-related quality of life, patient satisfaction, complications, re-operation, and healthcare resource use (such as length of stay) (13). Other knee outcomes had a similar pattern of small numerical, but not statistically significant, differences in favour of partial knee replacement. Length of stay, two of the three patient satisfaction outcomes, and a measure of overall health-related quality of life (score out of 100 by the participant) were statistically significantly higher in favour of partial knee replacement by a modest amount. Overall, both surgeries had similar high 5-year outcomes with similar clinical and surgical outcomes. Some small differences in favour of partial knee replacement in a patient-report measure of treatment approval were identified, which could be viewed as supporting partial knee replacement (all other things being equal).

In the LEAP trial, the overall result showed a strong effect in favour of consumption of peanuts. Secondary outcomes were occurrence of allergic sensitization, occurrence of food allergies, adverse events, and immunological assessments (14). Sensitization and immunological data also supported the overall conclusion. There were no deaths of study participants in the follow-up period. Hospitalization and serious adverse events were similar in the two groups. A key objective of the study was to explore whether the result was the same or not for the baseline SPT-positive and -negative groups. Corresponding analyses showed this was the case (in terms of favouring consumption though probably to a difference magnitude). Overall, the data provided a very convincing set of data in support of the consumption strategy.

In the IST trial, there were seven other pre-specified outcomes which included death or dependency at 6 months (a second primary outcome), and ischaemic stroke and major extracranial haemorrhage within 14 days, among others (8). A difference in favour of aspirin was observed in one of the key secondary outcomes (fewer ischaemic strokes within 14 days) with no increased risk of haemorrhagic strokes (considered a potential risk related to receipt of aspirin). Further analyses (including an analysis of death or dependency at 6 months adjusted for stroke severity at baseline) provided a consistent pattern of a small benefit with receipt of aspirin; hence the study's overall conclusion 'the IST suggests a small but worthwhile benefit [of aspirin] at 6 months'.

Other common issues in analysing clinical trial data

There are four key aspects of any clinical trial which need to be considered to make sure the analysis results are not misleading or at least no caveats need to be applied. These are (i) assessing the baseline comparability, (ii) the compliance with treatment allocation, (iii) the potential impact of missing data, and (iv) multiplicity of analyses. We consider each of these now in turn and use the three trials we considered above to consider the relevant issues.

Baseline comparability

When conducting a statistical analysis of an RCT, we wish to reassure ourselves that randomization was done as planned, and that there is no clear reason to doubt randomization has achieved what was intended. We have carried out randomization so that we have two groups that are comparable at baseline (at the point randomization occurred). As noted above, we wish to know that those analysed were those randomized. We can also check the key characteristics of the participants collected at the time of study entry prior to randomization to see that the randomized groups were indeed similar (22). This is called looking at baseline comparability. As noted earlier in Chapter 3, this requires more care than might at first appear to be the case, as randomization does not produce identical (perfectly 'matched') groups. Instead, with random allocation the groups are likely to be similar but we anticipate some chance differences. As such, if we have a number of characteristics we summarize at baseline, it would not be surprising for some to be a bit different. What we are looking for is extreme dissimilarity that might mean randomization was not carried out correctly. Or it would indicate that we have been extremely unfortunate in that randomization has produced groups which are clinically not comparable. Where stratification or minimization was used to control for one or more factors, we can check to see if the randomized groups are indeed very similar for thes factors which were controlled for. The randomization methods should have forced them to be similar. For example, if randomization was stratified by age, and age is very different in the two groups, it is a sign that randomization did not work as planned. It might indicate the randomization has been undermined. We can consider the TOPKAT trial again and note that the OKS at baseline was controlled for in the randomization. Looking at the baseline values in Table 9.1, we happily see that the mean (and standard deviation) of the OKS at baseline is very similar in both groups. This is as we would expect given the method of randomization used (minimization incorporating baseline OKS) and the size of the study. Happily, this is also true of the other two clinical factors (age and sex) which were included in the minimization algorithm (where 58% of participants were male in both groups and the average age was 65 SDs of 9) in both groups (13). In the LEAP trial, the randomization was stratified by SPT status at baseline. Of the 542 SPT-negative participants at baseline, 272 and 270 were in the consumption and avoidance groups, respectively. Similarly, of the SPT-positive participants, 51 and 47 were in the consumption and avoidance groups, respectively, suggesting the randomization worked as planned in this regard. Baseline characteristics were also reassuringly similarly (not shown here (14)) in the two groups.

Compliance with treatment allocation

We now consider the potential impact of compliance to the treatment allocation on the statistical analysis. Presuming randomization has been successful conducted, the trial has been appropriately conducted, and an appropriate statistical analysis has been conducted, then we have a valid result. However, to understand how it might be applied in clinical practice, or indeed if it has much value, we need to consider the compliance with treatment allocation. Did the participants allocated to a particular treatment receive it or not? If they did, was it received as planned? To give the extreme example, imagine if we had a study which found no difference between treatments in any outcomes. We would therefore think the choice of treatment makes no difference to the outcomes. However, if everyone actually got the same treatment (e.g. if everyone in the TOPKAT trial got total knee replacement) irrespective of randomization then observing no difference is hardly surprising. This is not telling us anything about a potential difference between total and partial knee replacement. It would also mean we have got something badly wrong with our trial design and conducting the trial. More likely, and what occurs in most clinical trials, is that most people receive what they were supposed to. However, we will have some who did not for various reasons. The magnitude of the proportion of non-compliance might make us reconsider our first interpretation.

For the TOPKAT trial, 88% of those in the partial knee replacement group actually got it, with 90% in the total knee replacement group getting a total knee replacement. Again, we have reassuringly large levels of compliance. Of note, though, there were 31 in the partial group who got a total knee replacement and 13 in the total group who got a partial knee replacement. This is sometimes called 'cross-over'. The impact of this is to dilute any genuine difference between the groups. For the LEAP trial the compliance data are reassuring: large differences in peanut consumption were found using a food questionnaire. Similarly, the level of peanut detected in bed dust samples also showed much more peanut consumption in the consumption group and little in the avoidance group as hoped (14). In the IST trial, we wish to consider whether the daily dose of aspirin was received for 14 days (unless discharged from hospital as planned). In the IST trial, pleasingly over 90% received their allocated treatment (92% of those allocated to aspirin took it as requested and 93% of those allocated to avoid it did not take it). This reassuringly suggests no reason to be concerned. Indeed, this might suggest a slightly higher benefit if aspirin is indeed taken.

Given this presence of some non-compliance in the TOPKAT, LEAP, and IST trials, it begs the question what would be the estimated treatment effect if treatment was fully received? This is a surprisingly difficult question to answer satisfactorily. A common approach is to compare only a subset of the randomized participants; under a 'per-protocol' analysis we only include in the analysis those allocated to each randomized group who have received the allocation as planned (i.e. allocated to aspirin and received aspirin). The advantage is that only those who got their allocated treatment are being compared. However, the disadvantage is that we have diluted the value of randomization by excluding a number of people from the randomized groups. This runs the risk of introducing selection bias when comparing these 'per-protocol' groups. For example, if more than one of the randomized group do not receive the full course of drug treatment because it has nasty side effects, those who drop out of the respective groups are likely to be different. The groups that are retained in the analysis accordingly may be a little different. A further fairly common approach is to analyse those as 'as treated', that is, ignoring the random allocations, and only focusing on what actually occurred, the key issue being that changing treatment will not be a random occurrence. It is usually related to the disease or general well-being (e.g. if they have more unwell). Both a per-protocol and an 'as-treated' analysis, are unsatisfactory ways to deal with non-compliance with random allocation. Fortunately, there are more sophisticated approaches to address this issue though they require careful implementation and interpretation. Complier-average causal effect methods to assess the causal effect in compliers have been used. The reader is referred to one of a number of excellent introductory texts for further information on their use in clinical trials and RCTs in particular (23). It is worth noting also that the cause of non-compliance is arguably as important as its existence in terms of the interpretation. Non-compliance with treatment allocation can unfortunately occur for study-related issues (e.g. the person delivering the treatment was unaware of the allocated intervention). However, it can also be for clinical reasons which might reflect use of the treatment in clinical practice (e.g. a drug may have a severe side effects in a minority of individuals). Any analysis seeking to address non-compliance requires careful interpretation. This also relates to what is the real research question of interest, and the analysis can be tailored to some degree to deal with the subtle nuances regarding compliance. The concept of 'estimands' is gaining in popularity in the statistical community as a way to express the analytic target more precisely, including how non-compliance and missing data should be dealt with (24). A ITT analysis as discussed above corresponds to a treatment policy estimand. Further discussion (24), of what can be quite complex subject is beyond the scope of this chapter; we note only here that the corresponding estimand analyses enviably have a trade-off of great assumptions to provide more tailored and specific results.

Dealing with missing data

Another key aspect of the statistical analysis is the strategy to address any missing data. Regrettably, the occurrence of missing outcome data seems unavoidable except for the smallest of clinical trials or where outcomes are restricted to those which are more readily collected (e.g. death or hospitalization). Similar to non-compliance, the presence of missing data may cause some uncertainty about the applicability of the result, and there is typically no entirely satisfactory analysis option. However, unlike non-compliance where some non-compliance may reflect clinical practice, missing data is purely a study issue. Therefore, in principle it can at least be mitigated and in some cases avoided by careful study design. Steps to minimize missing data particularly for key outcomes should be implemented. However, when it gets to the point when the statistical analysis is to be conducted, despite the hard work of many, having some missing key outcome data is far from uncommon. To consider the potential risk of bias we can quantify the magnitude of missing data by treatment groups. Hopefully, it is of a similarly low level in both groups so as not to be of any concern. For the LEAP trial, there were only 12 participants with missing primary outcome data (2%) (Table 9.2). This was 5 and 7 participants, respectively, in the consumption and avoidance groups. However, given the strength of the overall finding this is not of a magnitude that is overly concerning. No complex statistical method is needed to clarify this. In the IST study there were only two individuals (one in each group) missing 14-day data out of over 19,000 participants (Table 9.3). Clearly, missing data was also not a concern in this trial. In many settings, particularly patient-reported outcome, a substantial amount of missing data are unavoidable. There is no need to carry out any further analysis in this case. For example, in the TOPKAT trial the 5-year OKS was available for 88% and 89% of participants in the partial and total knee replacement groups, respectively. As 17 had died and a further 15 had withdrawn from the study by 5 years, the response rate (among those sent the questionnaire) was actually 92% and 95% in the partial and total knee replacement groups, respectively (11). Therefore, the amount of missing data was reassuringly small and similar in each group. However, we might still wish to carry out analyses to look at the impact involving 'imputation' to assess the potential impact. Methods to do so vary in complexity from one-off (e.g. 'simple' best–worse imputation for a binary outcome) to modelling potential outcomes based upon known data. Modelling approaches include 'multiple imputations' methods where multiple artificial datasets are generated with data imputed according to model assumptions. These datasets are then analysed individually and a summary result is produced, which is hopefully a fairer representation of the data.

It is worth noting that the presence of missing data per se does not invalidate the analysis even if there is a very high proportion (say, even 50%). However, the issue is whether having missing data has led to a biased analysis (due to the observed data not being representative of the complete dataset). Depending upon what view we take of the reasons for having missing data, we may be more or less concerned. If it is due to what statisticians would call 'missing completely at random' (unrelated to any patient characteristics) then having missing data will not bias the result. It will only reduce its precision. Similarly, if data are 'missing at random' (unrelated to patient characteristics as before once you take into account key information included in the analysis, e.g. sex and age at baseline) this can also be addressed in the analysis. We need the relevant data and to know what to adjust for. However, if the missing data are what is called 'missing not at random', then the presence of missing data makes the observed data unrepresentative. It therefore may lead to a biased analysis. When we are comparing between groups in an RCT, we have protection given the controlled nature of the groups. This is the case as long as the mechanism (factors) driving missing data is the same in both groups. However, this may not be the case. For example, if those in the group receiving one drug are more likely to leave the study and not provide outcome data due to adverse responses cause by that drug, then the impact of missing data could be just as bad in an RCT as in other studies. Often it is hard or impossible to be sure why data are missing. We might therefore want to think about how different the missing data might have to be from the observed data to make any difference to the conclusion we would draw from the results. All approaches to missing data, including acting as if there are none, make assumptions (explicitly or implicitly). Unfortunately these assumptions are largely uncheckable. Given this, a sensible approach is to quantify missing data, consider the reasons for it, and make use of analyses that can help explore its potential impact to alter the analysis result where it is non-negligible. Further details on dealing with missing data in clinical trials and the various missing approaches can be found elsewhere (25,26).

Dealing with multiplicity of analyses

We should also consider the potential for multiplicity of analyses when planning and conducting a statistical analysis. Often, for very good reasons, we have the potential for multiple analyses of in essence the same thing. We might measure an outcome, for example, in the TOPKAT trial the OKS was measured each year (e.g. 1, 2, 3, 4, and 5 years) and not just at 5 years. There may be different knee scores that could be used and collected in the trial. Furthermore, we could have a number of analyses to address the impact of missing data, compliance, or to use these data in different ways. For example, it might be believed that there could be an early difference in outcome but not at 5 years, or vice versa. There may be patient characteristics that might be considered to potentially affect how well the treatment works. These could be used to form subgroups of interest in which any differences in results could be explored. In the LEAP trial, the treatment effects in the SPT-positive and SPT-negative groups were of interest. Analysing these separately we have two analyses and two results (not one). If we also analyse the data overall (as we did earlier in the chapter), we can have three sets of results. More complex designs can also lead to multiple possible analyses (e.g. if we have three or more treatment groups we have seven possible analyses for each outcome). Very quickly we can tally up the analyses leading easily to double figures. As we noted above, there is nothing wrong per se with having multiple analyses. However, there is first the potential for additional analyses to provide a confusing and potentially contradictory array of results, and furthermore each additional analysis runs the risk of a spurious (i.e. not a genuine discovery but a unreliable) finding.

Formal statistical adjustment for such 'multiplicity' can be done which penalizes every statistical analysis carried out in order to preserve overall control on the possibility of a false finding (e.g. controlling the overall type I error) (27). However, these methods can be quite difficult to implement. They often require information that is not usually available upfront. Or they may be complex to abide by in practice when analysing and interpreting the results. The simplest approach, and the most commonly used, is the Bonferroni adjustment. Using this, the significance level is reduced by dividing the overall desired significance level by the number of statistical analyses considered to be related. For example, if in the LEAP trial we wanted to do separate analyses for the SPT-positive and SPT-negative baseline groups (and not analyse overall), we could carry out separate analyses by applying a 2.5% (5% divided by two) two-sided significance level to interpret the findings of the two analysis results (by adjusting the confidence interval accordingly). However, this approach is overly conservative in that it overcompensates. This approach quickly makes analyses fairly worthless as the number of analyses grows. Its impact can be compensated for by correspondingly substantially increasing the sample size but there is only so much of such inflation of the sample size that is possible. A better approach is to be clear what the planned main analysis is, and specify it as such. We then support this main result by choosing a small number of further analyses in advance which have a clear rationale. Other unplanned analyses which seem appropriate once the statistical analysis has begun can be marked as 'post hoc' when reporting (see Chapter 10 for more discussion). Doing so allows the reader to appropriately downplay the importance of the individual result. To summarize, when it comes to the analyses of each outcome, in general, less is more informative.

Analysis methods for other types of clinical trials

In the text so far we have considered the statistical analysis of RCTs. All comparative clinical trials will follow similar approaches though the outcomes considered and the analysis methods may differ. A very different class of clinical trials are early phase (1 and 2) clinical trials. These focus on safety consideration and early signs of treatment effect. In terms of the statistical analysis, typically evaluation of the safe dose (e.g. MTD) is commonly the main focus of these trials. Here the statistical design in terms of the sample size and analysis needs to be considered in light of the primary research question. For trials with dynamic dose-escalation, instead of a single analysis at the end which was implicitly assumed in the earlier discussion in this chapter, data will be analysed repeatedly as the study progresses. This is done in order to determine what the next dose should be or if the study can stop due to already reaching a conclusion according to the planned analysis. Modelling the PK and PD relationship might then be the focus in the final analysis in order to assess the recommended dose to use in a future study (e.g. phase 2 trial). The interested reader is referred to sources which deal with such analyses at some length (23,28–30).

Summary

The statistical analysis strategy should be tailored to the research objectives (reflecting their relative importance), the clinical trial design, the outcomes to be analysed, and the data to be collected. The more effort that is put into thinking about the statistical analysis in advance, the easier the process of analysing the trial will be. A main analysis should be specified for each outcome. Use of further (sensitivity and secondary) analyses can be helpful to tease out potential issues, nuances in interpretation, or provide reassurance related to assumptions. The potential impact of missing data and non-compliance should be explored. Nevertheless, the interpretation of these further results needs careful handling.

References

1. Stone GW, Pocock SJ. Randomized trials, statistics, and clinical inference. Journal of the American College of Cardiology. 2010;55(5):428–31.

2. Bland M. An Introduction to Medical Statistics. Oxford: Oxford University Press; 2015.
3. Kirkwood BR, Sterne JAC. Essential Medical Statistics. 2nd ed. Oxford: Blackwell Science; 2003.
4. Bland JM, Altman DG. Comparisons against baseline within randomised groups are often used and can be highly misleading. Trials. 2011;12(1):264.
5. Kahan BC, Jairath V, Doré CJ, Morris TP. The risks and rewards of covariate adjustment in randomized trials: an assessment of 12 outcomes from 8 studies. Trials. 2014;15:139.
6. Tsiatis AA, Davidian M, Zhang M, Lu X. Covariate adjustment for two-sample treatment comparisons in randomized clinical trials: a principled yet flexible approach. Stat Med. 2008 October 15;27(23):4658–4677. doi:10.1002/sim.3113
7. Senn S. Two cheers for P-values? Journal of Epidemiology and Biostatistics. 2001;6(2):193–204.
8. International Stroke Trial Collaborative Group. The International Stroke Trial (IST): a randomised trial of aspirin, subcutaneous heparin, both, or neither among 19435 patients with acute ischaemic stroke. Lancet. 1997;349(9065):1569–81.
9. Vickers AJ. Parametric versus non-parametric statistics in the analysis of randomized trials with non-normally distributed data. BMC Medical Research Methodology. 2005;5:35.
10. Cook JA, Julious SA, Sones W, Hampson LV, Hewitt C, Berlin JA, et al. Practical help for specifying the target difference in sample size calculations for RCTs: the DELTA(2) five-stage study, including a workshop. Health Technology Assessment. 2019;23(60):1–88.
11. Berry SM. Bayesian Adaptive Methods for Clinical Trials. Boca Raton, FL: Chapman & Hall/CRC; 2010.
12. Spiegelhalter DJ, Abrams KR, Myles JP. Bayesian Approaches to Clinical Trials and Health-Care Evaluation. Chichester: John Wiley & Sons; 2004.
13. Beard DJ, Davies LJ, Cook JA, MacLennan G, Price A, Kent S, et al. Total versus partial knee replacement in patients with medial compartment knee osteoarthritis: the TOPKAT RCT. Health Technology Assessment. 2020;24(20):1–98.
14. Du Toit G, Roberts G, Sayre PH, Bahnson HT, Radulovic S, Santos AF, et al. Randomized trial of peanut consumption in infants at risk for peanut allergy. New England Journal of Medicine. 2015;372(9):803–13.
15. Sackett DL, Deeks JJ, Altman DG. Down with odds ratios! Evidence Based Medicine. 1996;1(6):164.
16. Senn S. Odds ratios revisited. Evidence Based Medicine. 1998;3(3):71.
17. Newcombe RG. Interval estimation for the difference between independent proportions: comparison of eleven methods. Statistics in Medicine. 1998;17(8):873–90.
18. StataCorp. Stata: Release 15 [Statistical software]. College Station, TX: StataCorp; 2017.
19. Deeks JJ. Issues in the selection of a summary statistic for meta-analysis of clinical trials with binary outcomes. Statistics in Medicine. 2002;21(11):1575–600.
20. Stensrud MJ, Hernán MA. Why test for proportional hazards? JAMA. 2020;323(14):1401–2.
21. Jachno K, Heritier S, Wolfe R. Are non-constant rates and non-proportional treatment effects accounted for in the design and analysis of randomised controlled trials? A review of current practice. BMC Medical Research Methodology. 2019;19(1):103.
22. Altman DG. Comparability of randomised groups. Journal of the Royal Statistical Society Series D (The Statistician). 1985;34(1):125–36.
23. Senn S. Statistical Issues in Drug Development. 2nd ed. Chichester: John Wiley & Sons; 2007.
24. Rosenkranz S. Estimands—new statistical principle or the emperor's new clothes? Pharmaceutical Statistics. 2017;16:4–5.
25. Bell ML, Fiero M, Horton NJ, Hsu CH. Handling missing data in RCTs; a review of the top medical journals. BMC Medical Research Methodology. 2014;14:118.

26. Dziura JD, Post LA, Zhao Q, Fu Z, Peduzzi P. Strategies for dealing with missing data in clinical trials: from design to analysis. Yale Journal of Biology and Medicine. 2013;86(3):343–58.
27. Bender R, Lange S. Adjusting for multiple testing—when and how? Journal of Clinical Epidemiology. 2001;54(4):343–9.
28. Brown S, Gregory WM, Twelves C. A Practical Guide to Designing Phase II Trials in Oncology. Chichester: John Wiley & Sons; 2014.
29. Eisenhauer EA, Twelves C, Buyse M. Phase I Cancer Clinical Trials: A Practical Guide. 2nd ed. New York: Oxford University Press; 2015.
30. Julious SA, Machin D, Tan SB. An Introduction to Statistics in Early Phase Trials. Oxford: Wiley-Blackwell; 2010.

10

Reporting and disseminating the findings of a clinical trial

A high standard must be set in reporting the results of clinical trials, particular, as Daniels (1950) suggests, in these 'pioneering investigations' which 'may in many ways serve as a model and lesson to future investigators'.

Bradford Hill, 1951 (1)

Why reporting and dissemination matters

Reporting the results of a clinical trial can feel like a chore, a dull, if necessary, part of running a clinical trial. However, the value of good reporting cannot be overestimated. There are two main reasons why reporting matters.

First, those who conduct clinical trials have a moral obligation to report the findings so that others can benefit from their study. Regardless of the question a trial asks—learning about a new drug treatment, discovering the appropriate, safe dose of a drug, or seeing whether a new treatment is better than an alternative treatment—that question is not truly answered until the findings are reported to someone. Preferably they should be reported to many people and in different ways. Clinical trials impose obligations on those who take part. They may also expose participants to a higher risk than in typical clinical care, such as a first in human phase 1 clinical trial of a drug that has never been used in humans. There is little doubt that participants join trials at least partly because the study's result will be useful for someone. Arguably, a researcher's moral obligations towards the participants of research studies they run are only met when the findings are publicly and openly reported.

Second, reporting clinical trials helps prevent unnecessary or suboptimal treatment or experimentation on future patients and members of the public. If we discover that a drug does not work, or even causes harm, but we do not tell others, it is as if the study did not happen. In fact, it is even worse, as harm could have been avoided. We do not just need to report our findings—we need to report them as soon as possible.

Beyond these ethical reasons for adequate, timely reporting, there are also practical problems associated with poor reporting (2). Overviews of studies on a topic rely on being able to find every relevant study conducted. They may draw incorrect conclusions if published studies differ from those that remain unpublished—and indeed, 'negative' or disappointing studies (to some investigators, and some others) are less likely to be published. Even when published, research articles often fail to provide many basic pieces of information. This incomplete reporting can prevent a fair assessment of a study. How an RCT is designed and conducted can substantially alter the trustworthiness of its findings, as bias can be introduced at every stage in the trial's lifecycle. Readers cannot judge the reliability of findings without adequate reporting of important details. Unclear reporting can also obscure the implications of the study's findings. We need study details to determine whether a treatment worked, for whom this was shown, and how the treatment was given. Inadequate reporting can therefore lead to misallocation of future research funding, duplication of effort, and other forms of unnecessary research waste. It can hide the existence of datasets that could be used for other valid research purposes. It can also lead to clinical care that does not reflect the latest discoveries, causing preventable harm to patients.

Reporting is thus a key scientific endeavour for all research, but particularly for clinical trials given their relevance to patient care.

What is poor or inadequate reporting?

Clinical trial reporting can be inadequate even if the study and its main result are reported in an academic journal (2). Table 10.1 lists some common problems when reporting a trial and ways to prevent them (3–6).

We need to understand who the trial results might be relevant for. This requires clear reporting of who the research participants were and what happened to them. We also need to understand how the trial was conducted, how the data were collected, and what definitions were used. The data collected needs to be clearly reported, including how much there was, and what it looked like before analysis or analytic manipulation. This helps the reader to understand the results and use them in further research (e.g. a systematic review). Those involved in conducting systematic reviews are often frustrated by a lack of relevant data in study publications, making it impossible to work out whether the study should be included in an analysis, or to use it in a meta-analysis that combines data from multiple studies to produce an overall result.

The methods used in a clinical trial must be clearly stated. As we saw earlier, not all clinical trials are created equal. We need to know specific things about

Table 10.1 Common problems in how journal articles report clinical trial results and their remedies

Reporting inadequacy	Remedy
Failure to clearly identify the study design	• Register the clinical trial • Follow the CONSORT reporting guidelines (3) recommendations when naming the trial results article
Lack of key trial design details	• Follow the CONSORT reporting guidelines recommendations and relevant extensions when reporting key elements of trial design (e.g. randomization) in the trial results article
Inadequate intervention descriptions	• Use the SPIRIT (4), TIDIER (5), or other area-specific reporting guidelines (e.g. IDEAL framework for surgical interventions) (6)
Selective and misrepresentative reporting of outcome data	• Refer to trial registration and protocol documentation to ensure consistency or note and justify changes in the trial results article
Lack of clarity on treatment compliance	• Provide a CONSORT flow diagram in the trial results article • Report sufficient details in the article on what occurred and forms of non-compliance in the trial results article
Lack of clarity on presence of missing data	• Follow the CONSORT reporting guidelines recommendations and explicitly state how missing data were dealt with in the formation of groups and in the analysis in the trial results article
Insufficient reporting of outcomes to allow assessment of the magnitude of effect	• Make the clinical trial dataset available (e.g. in a data repository) • Provide summary data in the trial results article • Use analyses that quantify the magnitude of the effect size and associated uncertainty when analysing trial outcomes
Insufficient outcome data to allow incorporation in reviews and meta-analyses for comparison with other studies	• Make the clinical trial dataset available (e.g. in a data repository) • Use supplementary material to include necessary details that do not fit in the main text • Respond to queries from researchers seeking to use data
P-hacking	• Register the trial and clarify the study's primary objective and outcome in the registration entry • Specify analyses in a statistical analysis plan
Spin in interpretation	• Ask trial committee members to independently review the trial results • Solicit peer review of the trial results article and other outputs by publishing

the study to assess what was done and the associated risk of bias. The results of any data analysis, statistical or otherwise, should be reported and summarized in an accessible way.

Authors are also obligated to set their findings in the context of previous research. Ideally, authors would update a systematic review of the previous studies on this topic by including their new study. At the very least, authors should refer to key literature, including any existing systematic reviews and their findings and any landmark studies.

Good reporting is hard work

In most area of working life a pedantic colleague can be frustrating and might be best avoided. When it comes to reporting research studies, pedantic tendencies are virtuous, particularly for long-running, hard-to-conduct studies like clinical trials. For many clinical trials, the study team will be tired by the time they get to the point of reporting, some fed up with even the name of the study. Yet the hard work of reporting still needs to be done before the trial is truly complete, or we risk wasting all the hard work that has gone before. Reporting, even good reporting, generally goes unrecognized. People who are precise and insistent on clear and careful reporting, within reason and as long as they do not prevent reporting, thus serve a very useful role.

An example of a trial with clear and adequate reporting in the academic journal article is given in Table 10.2 (7). The Preloading trial was a two-arm, pragmatic trial that evaluated using a nicotine replacement before attempting to quit smoking ('preloading'). All the key elements we require to understand the basic design of the study were provided as shown in Table 10.2. We can readily see that the control arm had no active intervention. However, the lack of a true placebo, which might have been preferable, was noted by the investigators in the methods and discussion section. Prolonged abstinence from smoking, with a 2-week grace period, was stated to be the key (primary) outcome of interest, assessed at 6 months. Secondary outcomes were abstinence at 4 weeks and 12 months and biologically confirmed abstinence over a 7-day period, assessed at the different time points. From the details reported we can see the study had a coherent design to address the research question of interest.

In one regard at least, the reporting and specification could have been better. Although the study had a clearly specified primary analysis method, different results were produced from the model (OR, RR, and a risk difference). It was not clear which was the main result, and how any disagreement might be dealt with. Happily, all three effect measure estimates (OR, RR, and risk difference) had similar results in terms of statistical significance. Although only two of the three estimates were stated in the text shown in Table 10.2, the other was reported in one of the article's tables. The results

Table 10.2 Reporting key trial information—text from the Preloading smoking cessation trial

Element	Example text
Title	'Effects on abstinence of nicotine patch treatment before quitting smoking: parallel, two-arm, pragmatic randomised trial'
Objective	'To examine the effectiveness of a nicotine patch worn for four weeks before a quit attempt'
Population	'In three recruitment centres, based in Nottingham, Birmingham, and Bristol, general practitioners spoke or wrote to, emailed, or texted patients listed as smokers on the electronic health record and invited them to join the trial as a means to stop smoking'
Intervention	'We asked participants in the preloading arm to use a 21 mg/24 h nicotine patch daily for approximately 4 weeks before quit day'
Control	'We aimed to balance participants' expectations of success and to assess adverse events in an unbiased way. A placebo would have achieved this but owing to funding restrictions we developed a behavioural intervention. We asked participants to consider their smoking pattern, to consider the triggers for use of particular cigarettes, and to plan ways to reduce these cues'
Outcomes	'The primary outcome was prolonged biochemically validated abstinence measured six months after quitting The secondary outcomes were Russell standard abstinence at four weeks and 12 months, and biochemically confirmed seven day point prevalence abstinence at four weeks and six and 12 months'
Methods—design	'This was an open label multicentre pragmatic superiority trial, with participants randomised 1:1 to receive or not receive a nicotine patch to use for four weeks before quit day'
Methods—sample size	'Based on data from similar trials we estimated that 15% of participants in the control arm would achieve abstinence at six months We thought that a relative risk of 1.4 was both plausible and valuable for patients, implying a 6% absolute difference. This gave us a sample size of 893 in each study arm or 1786 in total, to achieve 90% power using χ^2 test with Yates's correction'
Methods—primary outcome	'The primary outcome was prolonged abstinence at six months, defined by the Russell standard criteria'
Methods—analysis population	'We followed the Russell standard approach to perform an intention to treat analysis for the abstinence outcome. Everyone randomised was included in the denominator, whenever and however smoking abstinence was assessed, and they were presumed to be smoking if this information was unknown'

(continued)

Table 10.2 Continued

Element	Example text
Methods—analysis method	'In the primary analysis, we calculated adjusted odds ratios using multivariable logistic regression in Stata 14.2 adjusted for the stratification variable (centre). We also calculated the percentage of participants achieving abstinence, the risk difference and risk ratios and 95% confidence intervals using the post-estimation adjrr procedure in Stata v14.2'
Results—primary outcome	'Biochemically validated abstinence at six months, was achieved by 157/899 (17.5%) of participants in the preloading arm and 129/893 (14.4%) in the control arm: a difference of 3.0% (95% confidence interval −0.4% to 6.4%); odds ratio 1.25 (95% confidence interval 0.97 to 1.62), P = 0.08 in the primary analysis'
Discussion	'In this pragmatic open label trial, there was no strong evidence that four weeks of nicotine patch treatment increased the rate of prolonged abstinence at six months in the primary analysis'
Conclusion	'Nicotine preloading with a 21 mg/24 h nicotine patch for four weeks seems to be efficacious, safe, and well tolerated, but probably deters the use of varenicline, the most effective smoking cessation drug'

of the main analysis of the primary outcome, frustratingly for the investigators, did not meet the pre-specified standard two-sided 5% significance level. Secondary outcomes analyses were reported and had similar results. A sensitivity analysis (noted to be pre-planned) adjusting for varenicline prescribed 1 week post-quit (30% in the control group versus 22% in the intervention group) was significant at all time points. Adverse events were reported and were similar in both groups. The discussion was similarly well written and began with the primary outcome result, reflecting the failure to show an effect even though one is plausible given the results. The final summary conclusion took into account the other outcomes and further analyses. Overall, the researchers suggested the treatment 'seems to be efficacious' but 'probably' also reduced the use of another treatment that is known to work. This interpretation hinged on the weight given to the secondary and sensitivity analyses that sought to deal with the presence of a non-trial treatment. The sensitivity analysis could have introduced bias rather than removing it as it adjusted for a post-randomization factor. Overall, the study was well reported and provided key information which enabled to reader to understand the study, what was done, and the interpretation of the investigator to make their own judgement.

Disseminating trial results

Start early

Dissemination of trial findings cannot be left to the end of the trial, as the groundwork for effective dissemination needs to be laid before the results are available. At the simplest level, this is done by making the relevant stakeholder groups and key decision-makers aware of the study's existence. Academic and industry studies can be funded in relative isolation from the health professionals who might alter their practice based on the findings. Decision-makers, whether regulatory or commissioners of care, similarly need to be made aware of the study and its findings. Some means of attracting their attention or reminding them periodically of the study is therefore needed. Communication must be kept going during the study to keep interested stakeholders engaged and ready for the release of the trial findings.

An effective dissemination strategy requires a range of outputs targeting different audiences (Table 10.3). It may also require engagement with key gatekeepers, such as professional societies, regulatory bodies like the MHRA and the FDA, and commissioners of care via relevant communities and representatives. Trial registration at the time of set-up is a key step in making a trial visible to others, as well as providing a means for others to assess the final trial against what was planned. Registering the study early on a suitable clinical trial registry is a key step in dissemination. Registries vary in the level of information required and which will be make publicly available. Basic information about the aim and basic design of the study, along with contract details, trial status, and related publications are basic requirements. Varying level of support for including trial results are provided on different registries. Some of the more commonly used registries are ClinicalTrials.gov, ISRCTN, and the EU clinical trials register (8–10). Clinical trials should be registered at the outset and preferably before recruitment begins. Updating the registry to provide the results when available may even be a legal requirement as it is in the US.

As well as direct contact and submissions to these groups, a study website and social media accounts can help with general awareness of the study. A good website can also be the means by which participants can be updated about the progress of the study and staff involved in the study can access key study documents and the database. Interested researchers may also view the study website. If the groundwork is done early, these means of communication will be much more effective as there will be an existing audience to talk to when the results are ready.

Table 10.3 Audience and principal communication methods

Principal audience	Form of communication
Potential participants and anyone who might be able to help identify them, such as health professionals	• Website • Email • Trial newsletters • Trial group meeting for the unveiling of the trial results • Presentations at professional group meetings (e.g. conference) • Media pieces (where the study area is particularly topical or the patient group is a substantial segment of the public population) • Relevant patient advocacy/support groups
Research community	• Trial registration • Journal articles (protocol, statistical analysis plan, trial results, etc.) • Presentations at professional group meetings (e.g. conferences) • Trial website
Health professional communities	• Journal articles (protocol, statistical analysis plan, trial results, etc.) • Presentations at professional group meetings (e.g. conferences) • Trial website
Members of the public and patients with relevant conditions and diseases (but not necessarily eligible to be a participant)	• Press release • TV, radio interviews • Lay summary • Podcasts • Blog posts • Social media • Visual abstracts (accessible graphical representations of the results) • Video presenting the trial findings in an accessible manner • Public engagement events (e.g. in partnership with relevant patient advocacy group)
Trial participants	• Participant newsletters • Personalized/generic emails • Moderated social media groups • Video presenting the trial to potential participants

Perhaps less important than in the past, but still a key part of disseminating trial results, is presenting the trial progress and results at academic conferences and professional special interest meetings. In the past, results were often unveiled for the first time at these groups. Increasingly, these meetings offer an accessible introduction to the study and its findings and a signpost to the academic trial results article and other dissemination resources such as the website and social media. This is particularly true as the length of conference presentations have shortened in recent years (e.g. 10 minutes), and there is so much information relevant to the trial to provide.

The publication in an academic journal of the trial results is still the key moment in the dissemination of trial results. However, we also need a range of different outputs to reach all relevant audiences. Many journals now include bullet-point lists and plain language summaries alongside traditional abstracts to increase accessibility. Social media, particularly Twitter, is also increasingly part of the process used by funders, journals, investigators, and their institutions to try to pique the interest of news outlets, along with more traditional press releases.

Different audiences and different means of communication

Traditionally, clinical trials have generally had a single key audience. For academic-led studies it was the clinical community which was typically reached by publishing an article reporting the study in an academic journal. The article should be published in a PubMed-indexed journal (11). Doing so ensures multiple formats (title and abstract only, and the full article) are produced and disseminated via multiple means (e.g. the journal's website and social media accounts, title and abstract on PubMed and potentially other medical databases). PubMed-indexed journals are those where the title and abstract of each published article will be included in the online PubMed database. Searching the PubMed database has become a quick, freely accessible, and indispensable way for researchers and health professionals to identify relevant research articles. In addition to the journal article, a conference presentation or two might be made at the relevant medical society meeting either before or after the paper is published. In industry-sponsored phase 1 or 2 trials, it is the internal senior management who are the target audience. The aim is to inform the commercial and scientific decision of whether to proceed with the drug to the next phase of development. For industry-sponsored phase 3 trials, it is regulatory bodies via a regulatory submission, prepared by the sponsoring company.

While these are still arguably the key audiences for these types of clinical trials, all clinical trials must also communicate information about themselves to multiple audiences using appropriate means. This reflects increasing recognition of the limitations in what the primary means of communication achieve by themselves. It also reflects the need to cater to multiple audiences, and changes in legal requirements, and expectations of professional and research communities. For example, expectations around communication with the public have markedly changed. It is now common for large phase 3 trials to provide accessible summaries to patients as the study progresses, and to summarize the results in 'Plain English language'.

A key change in dissemination findings over the last 10 years has been how quickly articles can appear in the public domain. No longer are journals the only way, as long as someone has a sufficiently large social media presence results can be shared quickly and widely. Most large institutions, such as universities, colleges, and companies, have a dedicated communications team ready to help promote the findings of a study. This is often done via a short summary of a study's findings and, for particularly noteworthy trials, their initiation and updates. A press release might accompany this, particularly for noteworthy findings. Such promotional materials need to be accessible to the public to attract attention and facilitate re-use. However, no matter how exciting the study and its findings, social media promotions only work when backed up by other means of communications. They are typically timed for the unveiling of findings at a clinical conference, or the publication of an article reporting the results. A full version of the study results should be available to provide more information to accompany a press release. This will help address the inevitable queries that arise about how the trial was conducted and further data, and would typically be raised by the release of the result. Ideally the press release is arranged to coincide with the publication of the results article.

Open access publication is also increasingly important. Articles published as open access are freely available to read for all, irrespective of where readers are located and whether they have access to a personal or institutional journal subscription. Open access publication usually requires the author to pay an article processing charge after acceptance. More established and prestigious traditional journals tend to charge higher fees than others to make articles open access. Increasingly, public and charity research funders are requiring open access publication and are providing funding to deliver this.

In the past, there was often a long delay between an article being accepted for publication and it finally appearing in print. Many journals now publish an 'online-only' version of the article well ahead of their print version (if this exists). These online-only versions are still the final version of the article—they have been through peer review, accepted, and formatted to the journal's style. They may simply be missing the final article's full citation, which is only available once the 'print' issue is compiled.

Other journals have gone a step further and make available an earlier version of the manuscript. The 'postprint' or 'author accepted manuscript' is the version of the article after peer review and unconditional acceptance, but before the journal has applied its formatting. Journals share these 'accepted' manuscripts, often under the same digital object identifier that the final print version will hold. There is usually a caveat that the article may still be subject to small changes due to typesetting and proofing.

The practice of sharing preprints has recently become more common in the biomedical sciences. Here a version of the article is shared publicly before peer review begins. This approach is appealing when study findings are considered particularly time-sensitive. Some journals facilitate preprint sharing of the manuscripts submitted to them through their own platforms. Alternatively, authors can share their preprints in dedicated preprint servers that function completely separately from any academic journal, such as medRxiv (12). An article shared on a preprint server does not have to ever be submitted to a journal. Colleagues can review and provide comments on these manuscripts, again, unconnected to any journal, and authors can make rounds of revisions as they wish (13). Most journals do not consider sharing preprints on preprint servers to be prior publication. Authors therefore have the option to later, or even concurrently, submit to a journal. Using preprint servers in this way has become very common in some areas of sciences, such as physics and mathematics.

Clinical medicine has been slow to embrace preprints, possibly due to the wider array of audiences, the potential speed at which findings might be applied, and the potential for harm if a study has not been vetted by independent assessors. Nevertheless, a few recent high-profile trials have successfully used preprints. The most remarkable example was the preprint publication of the trial results article for the RECOVERY COVID-19 trial. The press release of the findings and the preprint article appeared before the formal academic publication of the findings. The preprint publication led to changes in clinical practice within days, before the formal publication of the results article in a medical journal occurred almost a month later (14). The preprint model may help to speed up the publication of key findings. It arguably leads to a better final publication, as many more people can review and comment than the handful of peer reviewers and editors involved in most traditional journal articles. However, it remains to be seen how much clinical trial publication practices will move in this direction. The potential for misunderstanding and misapplication is perhaps greater than in any other area of science. Additionally, clinical trials are very complex studies to report well. As such, the slower and multiple-stage process (away from the general release) has its benefits even if it does delay the release of important findings.

As well as the traditional means of publishing an academic article, and presentations to professional bodies, social media is increasingly used to promote clinical trials and to disseminate their findings. Along with this there is increasing interest in more accessible forms of presenting both an overview of the trial and the key findings of a trial. This includes forms such as visual abstracts (a type of infographic used to provide a graphical representation of trial findings) (15). Short videos which present the trial and/or its findings and can be shared on social media, and made available via the trial website (15). These can be developed with health professionals, patients, or members of the public in mind.

In the remainder of this chapter we will focus on the main output needed to effectively communicate trial results: the academic journal article reporting its main findings. We will also consider the merits of sharing the trial dataset.

Academic journal articles

The critical importance of reporting as part of the research endeavour was recognized back in the 1950s as a key step in the clinical trial process (1,16). Nevertheless, it is only in the last 10–20 years that the quality of reporting has perhaps received the attention it deserves. As the decades progressed, the value of clear and comprehensive reporting has become clearer, regrettably in its absence in an increasing proportion of studies. The complexity of clinical trials and the multifaceted nature of what needs to be reported has also become clearer. Different aspects of clinical trials have been explored methodologically and through reviews of published clinical trials have highlighted areas for improvement (2,17). Thankfully, standards of reporting seem to be rising, although they are still not what they ought to be (18).

Perhaps the most important step in improving reporting has been the creation of a clear and well-developed reporting guideline, the CONsolidated Standards of Reporting Trials (CONSORT) statement, in 1996 (3). Reporting guidelines are checklists, flow diagrams, or structured text to guide authors in reporting a specific type of research and aim to remind authors of the minimum information readers need. Although CONSORT focuses on RCTs, its impact has been felt on all clinical trials and beyond into almost all areas of medicine. It has inspired the creation of similar guidelines for reporting systematic reviews, cohort studies, and many other study designs and clinical areas.

CONSORT was updated in 2010, and a new update is in progress. The current CONSORT statement includes a 25-item checklist for reporting, along with a helpful companion explanation and elaboration article that explains why each item is needed and gives examples of good reporting from published papers. The checklist is reproduced in Table 10.4 (19). It covers the various sections of an article: title, abstract, background, methods, results, and discussion. It also covers key information important to understanding a trial, such as the availability of the study protocol and trial registration number. Many journals request authors of clinical trial results articles to adhere to CONSORT. Some require authors to indicate on a checklist on which page of their manuscript each item has been reported. The completed checklist is submitting alongside the trial results article as evidence of sufficient reporting.

A similar reporting guideline exists for RCT protocols (SPIRIT) (4) and interventions (TIDieR) (5). Many other standards exist for RCT-related aspects of reporting, such as the DELTA^2 statement for reporting sample size calculations (20). The EQUATOR Network provides an extensive list of reporting guidelines for all types of human health research studies (21).

The CONSORT statement also suggests that authors include a participant flow diagram in their manuscripts. This recommendation has been as important for ensuring adequate reporting as the full checklist. Building on previous figures used to illustrate earlier studies, it helpfully provides an overview of the study conduct and is often the easiest way to quickly understand the basic design and running of an RCT. The diagram neatly shows the flow of individuals. This starts with assessment for eligibility, to being approached to take part in the study, and then to being randomized and allocated to each treatment group. Within the treatment groups, the flow of participants and whether they receive or not the allocated intervention is given. Similarly, the available data at the key time points in participant follow-up and how people were included in the analysis is given for the randomized group.

An example CONSORT flow diagram is given in Figure 10.1 for the preloading example we considered earlier in this chapter (7). It clearly summarizes the assessment of eligibility and who eventually participated in the study. The number of participants in each randomized group as time progresses is shown. All participants are clearly accounted for at the primary outcome time-point (6 months). However, for some of the other time-points this is not the case. Clearly reporting data availability over multiple time-points is not straight-forward. Loss of contact with participants can be seen to grow over the follow-up time, with about 80% providing information at 6 and 12 months. Compliance data were reported separately in the text of the article, reflecting a modification to the basic flow diagram structure. The point being the information was made available in the article whether in the figure, in the text, or both.

A growing number of extensions to the main CONSORT statement have been developed to address additional needs for alternative trial designs (e.g.

Table 10.4 CONSORT 2010 list of reporting items

Section of article	Checklist item	Description
Tile and abstract	Identification	Identification as a randomized trial in the title
	Structured summary	Structured summary of trial design, methods, results, and conclusions (for specific guidance see CONSORT for abstracts)
Introduction	Background	Scientific background and explanation of rationale
	Objectives	Specific objectives or hypotheses
Methods	Trial design	Description of trial design (such as parallel, factorial) including allocation ratio
	Important changes	Important changes to methods after trial commencement (such as eligibility criteria), with reasons
	Participants: eligibility	Eligibility criteria for participants
	Participants: settings	Settings and locations where the data were collected
	Interventions	The interventions for each group with sufficient details to allow replication, including how and when they were actually administered
	Outcomes	Completely defined pre-specified primary and secondary outcome measures, including how and when they were assessed
		Any changes to trial outcomes after the trial commenced, with reasons
	Sample size: determination	How sample size was determined
	Sample size: interim analyses	When applicable, explanation of any interim analyses and stopping guidelines
	Randomization: sequence generation method	Method used to generate the random allocation sequence
	Randomization: type	Type of randomization; details of any restriction (such as blocking and block size)
	Randomization: allocation concealment	Mechanism used to implement the random allocation sequence (such as sequentially numbered containers), describing any steps taken to conceal the sequence until interventions were assigned
	Randomization: implementation	Who generated the random allocation sequence, who enrolled participants, and who assigned participants to interventions
	Blinding: summary	If done, who was blinded after assignment to interventions (e.g. participants, care providers, those assessing outcomes) and how
	Blinding: similarity	If relevant, description of the similarity of interventions
	Statistical methods: primary and secondary outcomes	Statistical methods used to compare groups for primary and secondary outcomes

Table 10.4 Continued

Section of article	Checklist item	Description
	Statistical methods: additional analyses	Methods for additional analyses, such as subgroup analyses and adjusted analyses
Results	Participant flow: randomized, complied, and analysed	For each group, the numbers of participants who were randomly assigned, received intended treatment, and were analysed for the primary outcome
	Participant flow: losses and withdrawal	For each group, losses and exclusions after randomization, together with reasons
	Recruitment: dates	Dates defining the periods of recruitment and follow-up
	Recruitment: stopping	Why the trial ended or was stopped
	Baseline data	A table showing baseline demographic and clinical characteristics for each group
	Numbers analysed	For each group, number of participants (denominator) included in each analysis and whether the analysis was by original assigned groups
	Outcomes and estimation	For each primary and secondary outcome, results for each group, and the estimated effect size and its precision (such as 95% confidence interval)
		For binary outcomes, presentation of both absolute and relative effect sizes is recommended
	Ancillary analyses	Results of any other analyses performed, including subgroup analyses and adjusted analyses, distinguishing pre-specified from exploratory
	Harms	All important harms or unintended effects in each group (for specific guidance see CONSORT for harms)
Discussion	Limitations	Trial limitations, addressing sources of potential bias, imprecision, and, if relevant, multiplicity of analyses
	Generalizability	Generalizability (external validity, applicability) of the trial findings
	Interpretation	Interpretation consistent with results, balancing benefits and harms, and considering other relevant evidence
Other information	Registration	Registration number and name of trial registry
	Protocol	Where the full trial protocol can be accessed, if available
	Funding	Sources of funding and other support (such as supply of drugs), role of funders

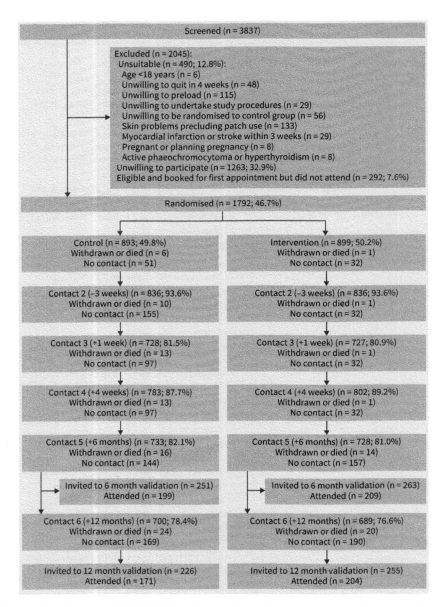

Figure 10.1 Example CONSORT flow diagram (from the Preloading smoking cessation trial) (7).

cluster trials), specific intervention types (e.g. non-drug treatments), and specific aspects of reporting (e.g. abstracts and harms) (3). If used appropriately alongside the main CONSORT statement, these extensions further enhance the reporting of the relevant aspects of trial design and conduct. While academic publication is a necessary step, it is not sufficient on its own. Increasingly the sharing of the corresponding data in some manner is required.

Making the data available

Many errors in reporting and statistical analysis can be identified in a transparently reported study. It is possible to identify fundamental problems in study design or even potential cases of scientific fraud from the trial results article alone (22). Other errors may not be readily identifiable and only if the reported results are particularly implausible or the model is clearly inappropriate, such as errors in the specification of a statistical model that uses three or more variables. Only independent verification of findings can give the final reassurance that there are no reproducibility issues. The sharing of trial data has therefore received increasing prominence over the last 10 years, particularly due to how easy electronic data transfer has become.

Sharing data has other benefits. Other researchers can produce the summary values they need, which may differ from those presented in the trial results paper. Systematic reviewers can conduct individual patient data analyses that fully utilize the potential information from included studies, rather than simpler analyses based on data summaries such as the number of people in each group and how many had an event. The robustness of the reported findings can be explored in greater detail than in the main analysis. Later research may raise a related research question not anticipated at the time of conducting the main trial analysis. Additional questions can be addressed beyond the work of the main paper. Datasets can also be used to evaluate research methodologies in real-world data rather than simulated data. They can also serve as examples as we have done with the IST and LEAP trials data in Chapter 9 both of which are available to anyone to access (23). This may be done via a data repository through which datasets from clinical trials like other studies can be made freely available (24).

Given these benefits, why are so few datasets made available for other researchers or interested parties? Clinical trials are planned experiments, and this planning should include their analysis as we have already noted. Making data available opens the study up to potential spurious findings, whether due to multiplicity of analyses or data misuse. As a consequence, many trial groups favour a 'controlled access' model of data sharing. Data are made available in response to reasonable requests, provided certain conditions are met, rather than making data freely available via an institutional or journal website, or via a data repository.

Clinical trials are also time-consuming, expensive endeavours. Those who have undertaken this burden have a natural sense of 'ownership' over the initial use of the data and are often best placed (at least in principle) to use it as they understand it better than anyone else. The trial team may have planned further secondary outputs. The timing of data sharing, whether the whole dataset or a portion, is therefore not clear in every case. When data are eventually shared and used, some method of recognition of those who undertook the original study seems appropriate. An acknowledgement in a future publication can seem like scant recognition for the hard slog of conducting the study which any secondary work is entirely dependent on.

Furthmore, publishing of data is hard work. It requires more documentation and clarity than otherwise might be needed. Data sharing requires care to ensure that only certain, non-identifiable data are shared. It is generally accepted that further sharing of the participant level data requires the express permission of the individuals concerned if there is any identifiable information. This implies a corresponding statement on any consent form, and in the protocol and any related ethical review submission. Restrictions on sharing data are often legally enforced via data protection laws (e.g. common law and the Data Protection Act 2018 in the UK) and governmental regulations. Fortunately, meeting these requirements is not an insurmountable issue, as the level of information from clinical trials that most potential users would like to have access to matches them. However, researchers cannot simply 'dump' all of the data from a study online. They must process and review the data to maintain the rights of those who took part, sometimes withholding certain data from sharing or converting data into a format that is less identifiable. For example, age (in years) could be shared but not date of birth. They may need to review hundreds or even thousands of variables. In some cases, someone will have to go through each individual's information for some data variables to ensure no personal data are accidently shared. Personal data may be sharable with others, provided they commit to maintaining these data securely, and appropriate permissions have been received. Shared data are typically anonymized to ensure no one is identifiable and explicit permission for the sharing is not required. Trials groups and institutions that sponsor research have developed systems and processes to ensure data are managed and processed appropriately, including secure sharing. However, this adds further work, often without dedicated time, funding, or professional recognition.

Nevertheless, expectations for data sharing have increased over the last 10 years. Some public sector and charity funders now insist on data being available for at least some purposes. Regulatory bodies may request access to the data, and journals may request independent assessment if the integrity of research findings are queried. Data sharing is now increasingly part of the reporting process and trialists should expect to share at least some part of their collected data. Some handy practical guidance on how to make clinical trial data are available, although local laws and institutional policies vary (25).

Summary

The reporting of clinical trials should be seen as an ethical imperative and a key step in the scientific process. Over the last 20 years, there has been a shift in the modes and mechanisms of reporting and how to engage with interested stakeholders and disseminate findings. Social media holds an increasing role in promotion, along with engagement with decision-makers. Making data available is also becoming more common, typically using a controlled access model. Clinical trial journal articles reporting the main results are the keystone of clinical trial reporting. From the scientific perspective, they are the foundation upon which other reporting and dissemination endeavours stand or fall. However, other forms of dissemination are increasingly important.

References

1. Hill AB. The clinical trial. British Medical Bulletin. 1951;7(4):278–82.
2. Glasziou P, Altman DG, Bossuyt P, Boutron I, Clarke M, Julious S, et al. Reducing waste from incomplete or unusable reports of biomedical research. Lancet. 2014;383(9913):267–76.
3. CONSORT group. Homepage. 2023. Available from: http://www.consort-statement.org/
4. SPIRIT Group. Guidance for clinical trials protocols. 2021. Available from: https://www.spirit-statement.org/
5. Hoffmann TC, Glasziou PP, Boutron I, Milne R, Perera R, Moher D, et al. Better reporting of interventions: template for intervention description and replication (TIDieR) checklist and guide. BMJ. 2014;348:g1687.
6. McCulloch P, Altman DG, Campbell WB, Flum DR, Glasziou P, Marshall JC, et al. No surgical innovation without evaluation: the IDEAL recommendations. Lancet. 2009;374(9695):1105–12.
7. The Preloading Investigators. Effects on abstinence of nicotine patch treatment before quitting smoking: parallel, two arm, pragmatic randomised trial. BMJ. 2018;361:k2164.
8. National Library of Medicine. ClinicalTrials.gov. 2023. Available from: https://clinicaltrials.gov/
9. BioMed Central Ltd. ISRCTN registry. 2022. Available from: https://www.isrctn.com/
10. European Medicines Agency. EU clinical trials register. 2021. Available from: https://www.clinicaltrialsregister.eu/

11. National Library of Medicine. PubMed.gov. 2023. Available from: https://pubmed.ncbi.nlm.nih.gov/

12. Cold Spring Harbor Laboratory. medRxiv: the preprint server for health sciences. 2023. Available from: https://www.medrxiv.org/

13. Rawlinson C. New preprint server for medical research. BMJ. 2019;365:l2301.

14. Mahase E. Covid-19: demand for dexamethasone surges as RECOVERY trial publishes preprint. BMJ. 2020;369:m2512.

15. FORCE study collaborators. The FORCE study. 2022. Available from: https://force-dissemination.digitrial.com/

16. Crofton J. Marc Daniels (1907–1953): a pioneer in establishing standards for doing and reporting clinical trials. Journal of the Royal Society of Medicine. 2014;107(2):79–81.

17. Boutron I, Guittet L, Estellat C, Moher D, Hróbjartsson A, Ravaud P. Reporting methods of blinding in randomized trials assessing nonpharmacological treatments. PLoS Medicine. 2007;4(2):e61.

18. Dechartres A, Trinquart L, Atal I, Moher D, Dickersin K, Boutron I, et al. Evolution of poor reporting and inadequate methods over time in 20 920 randomised controlled trials included in Cochrane reviews: research on research study. BMJ. 2017;357:j2490.

19. Schulz KF, Altman DG, Moher D. CONSORT 2010 statement: updated guidelines for reporting parallel group randomised trials. BMC Medicine. 2010;8:18.

20. Cook JA, Julious SA, Sones W, Hampson LV, Hewitt C, Berlin JA, et al. DELTA(2) guidance on choosing the target difference and undertaking and reporting the sample size calculation for a randomised controlled trial. BMJ. 2018;363:k3750.

21. The EQUATOR Network. Homepage. 2021. Available from: https://www.equator-network.org/

22. Bolland MJ, Gamble GD, Avenell A, Grey A. Identical summary statistics were uncommon in randomized trials and cohort studies. Journal of Clinical Epidemiology. 2021;136:180–8.

23. Sandercock PA, Niewada M, Członkowska A. The International Stroke Trial database. Trials. 2011;12:101.

24. Banzi R, Canham S, Kuchinke W, Krleza-Jeric K, Demotes-Mainard J, Ohmann C. Evaluation of repositories for sharing individual-participant data from clinical studies. Trials. 2019;20(1):169.

25. Keerie C, Tuck C, Milne G, Eldridge S, Wright N, Lewis SC. Data sharing in clinical trials—practical guidance on anonymising trial datasets. Trials. 2018;19(1):25.

Glossary of key clinical trial terms

Adaptive trial A type of clinical trial which uses a study design where specific adaptations to the study design part way through the conduct of the clinical trial are allowed for.

Adverse event An incident involving a participant in a clinical trial. Adverse events vary in their seriousness. Whether they are of an anticipated nature, thought to be related to the clinical trial, and specifically related to the treatments under evaluation are key attributes to consider.

Allocation concealment When there is no knowledge of future allocations. Maintaining allocation concealment requires the provision of the next allocation without revealing future allocations. It also requires the previous allocation to not reveal the next allocation. Different approaches can be used to ensure this. These include ensuring a different person generates the sequence (and has access to it) from the individual who recruits to the randomized controlled trial.

Bayesian statistics An approach to statistics which seeks to update prior evidence (belief) with the new data provided by the current study. It differs from the conventional (or frequentist) statistical approach in a number of key regards such as the need to explicitly quantify prior evidence, along with specifying how the existing information will be updated. The name comes from the Reverend Thomas Bayes who used a formula now known as Bayes theorem to update the probability of an event given new information.

Bias The tendency to produce an estimate which is not a fair reflection of the true state. In the context of clinical trials, it is an inclination to favour one treatment over the other which is not a true reflection of the respective effects of the treatments. Different sources of bias can exist. The presence of a source of bias does not necessarily mean the finding of a study is wrong.

Blinding The absence of knowledge of the treatment allocation given to participants. The term masking is often used to indicate the same thing. Different individuals involved in a randomized controlled trial can be blinded or not.

Clinical trial A planned scientific study involving human participants which is conducted to learn about the safety and 'efficacy' (i.e. positive medical effect) of a medical treatment or related care. Related care includes screening and use of diagnostic tests. The term 'clinical trials' like many academic terms has been used in various ways. At points it has been used to indicate any study evaluating a treatment. However, a narrower usage is more common, which is restricted to those with some prospective data collection to compare medical interventions (usually treatments). The term is now commonly applied to studies evaluating 'medical devices' as well as drugs and other treatments like surgery.

Confidence interval A range of values for the parameter of interest (e.g. mean difference) which contains the true value with the stated level of confidence. Confidence here refers to the desired percentage of times the true value is contained in the interval if the analysis were to be undertaken repeatedly (i.e. assuming random sampling). Typically, in a clinical trial, this confidence is set at the 95% level which corresponds to a two-sided 5% significance level (i.e. a 95% confidence interval is produced).

Control The treatment to which the intervention is intended to be compared. The control treatment can be a variety of different things including a placebo, alternative active treatment, current practice, or the absence of the intervention treatment.

CTIMP A clinical trial of an investigational medicinal product (IMP). To be a CTIMP, a clinical trial has to evaluate at least one IMP.

Follow-up The process by which the involvement of a participant in a clinical trial is tracked and relevant treatment, safety, and efficacy data are collected.

Informed consent Agreement to take part in a clinical trial from an individual who has sufficient understanding of the implications of taking part.

Intention to treat Grouping of the data in the statistical analysis in the way which reflects the randomization process when analysing a randomized controlled trial. It is the 'intent' to give the treatment, not the receipt of it, which is the determinant of the groups (i.e. groups are 'as randomized').

Interim analysis A formal statistical analysis conducted part way through the conduct of a clinical trial in order to make a key decision about the study's continuation.

Intervention The treatment which is being evaluated in the clinical trial. Typically, the intervention is a new treatment (e.g. a new drug) which is compared in the study to a control treatment.

Investigational medicinal product A drug which meets the legal regulatory definition of an Investigational Medicinal Product (IMP). This terminology is used in the UK and European Union member states. In the US, the corresponding terminology invoking regulatory implications is 'Investigational New Drug'. Elsewhere the terminology may be 'investigational' medicine, product, or drug.

Outcome A measure by which the effect of a treatment can be quantified. The outcomes collected in a trial can be subdivided into primary and secondary outcomes. The primary outcome is the one which the main research question most directly relates to. Other outcomes are classified as secondary outcomes. Outcomes in clinical trials may also be categorized according to whether they are considered to mainly relate to the efficacy or safety of the treatments.

Participant An individual involved in the clinical trial and for whom data will be collected and analysed. Typically, these individuals are patients with a condition for which the treatments are intended though this is not always the case.

Placebo An intervention which mimics a treatment being evaluated in a study but does not contain the active ingredient/critical element.

Population The group of interest to whom the evaluation pertains.

P-value The probability of a result as or more extreme than the one observed assuming the null hypothesis is true. The null hypothesis varies according to the framing of the study's research question. In the context of clinical trials, the null hypothesis is usually that there is no difference between the intervention and control (i.e. addressing a 2-sided superiority question). The p-value is one of a number of possible ways to summarize the findings from a statistical analysis.

Randomization The process by which a random treatment allocation is produced. Three main types of randomization exist: simple, restricted, and outcome-adaptive.

Randomized controlled trial A scientific study where the intervention and control (e.g. treatments) under evaluation are allocated to participants according to a random process. The name is often shortened to RCT.

Sample size The number of individuals involved in a clinical trial. Typically, a sample size calculation is carried out in advance to determine the number of individuals needed in order to provide reassurance that the study is likely to achieve its primary objective. Conventionally this is framed in terms of having sufficient statistical power given a set of assumptions related to the outcome data and planned statistical analysis, and a pre-specified statistical significance level.

Sequence generation The process by which the sequence of random allocations is generated for a randomized controlled trial. A variety of approaches could be used ranging from tossing a coin to automated telephone and webpage-based computer-generated allocation systems. The approach used has implications for the provision of the allocations, and also for allocation concealment.

Statistical power The probability that a difference of a pre-specified magnitude will be detected in the planned statistical analysis given a set of assumptions relating to the study design, outcome data and planned statistical analysis.

Statistical significance The term used to signify a level of statistical evidence relating to how unusual the observed data are given the statistical analysis carried out. It is conventionally defined by selecting a probability (alpha) level which is then applied to a statistical analysis result. For the result to be 'statistically significant', the p-value has to less or equal to this value. Typically, in a clinical trial this statistical significance level is set at 5% and a difference in either direction (two-sided, i.e. higher or lower in the intervention than the control group) is allowed for. Correspondingly, the $100 \times (1 - \text{alpha})\%$ confidence interval from the analysis of a randomized controlled trial would have to exclude the value of no difference (e.g. zero for a 95% confidence interval for the mean difference) for the result to be considered 'statistically significant'. Statistical significance does not necessarily imply that the finding has any clinical or practical significance. Such a judgement has to be based on consideration of the magnitude and object of interest (e.g. a X treatment effect in Y is viewed as important).

Study design The basic framework of the study. A randomized controlled trial is a specific type of study design of which there are a number of variations. Other types of clinical trials use different study designs.

Target difference The difference in the outcome of interest which the study sample size calculation is based upon. Various approaches can be used to determine the approach value to use including seeking to find the smallest value that is viewed as clinically important (e.g. minimum clinically important difference).

Index

For the benefit of digital users, indexed terms that span two pages (e.g., 52–53) may, on occasion, appear on only one of those pages.

Tables, and figures are indicated by an italic *t*, and *f* following the page/paragraph number.